Current Trends in Cancer Management

Edited by Liliana Streba, Dan Ionut Gheonea and Michael Schenker

Published in London, United Kingdom

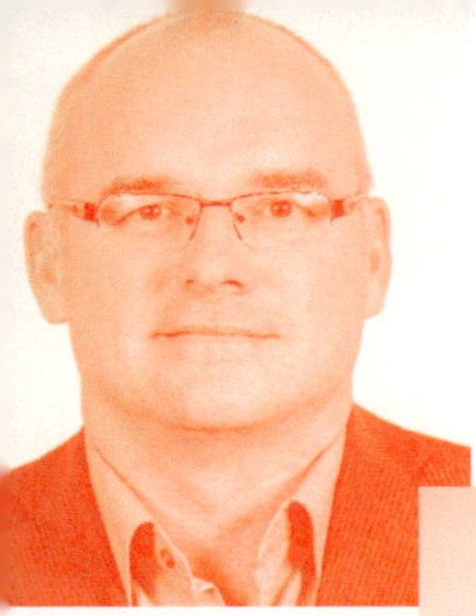
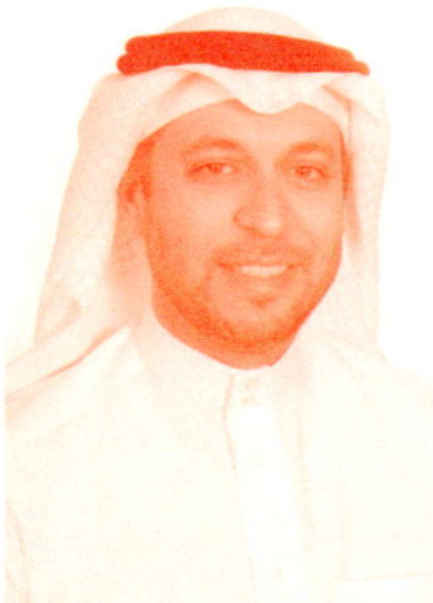
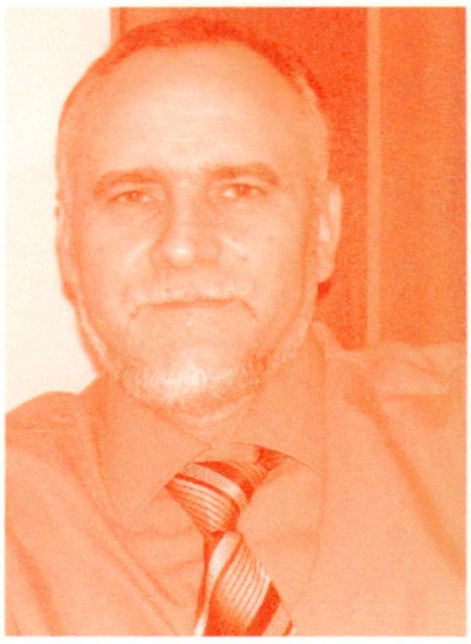
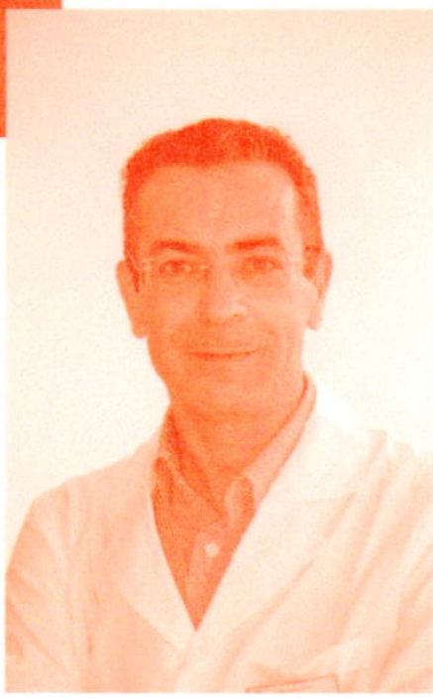
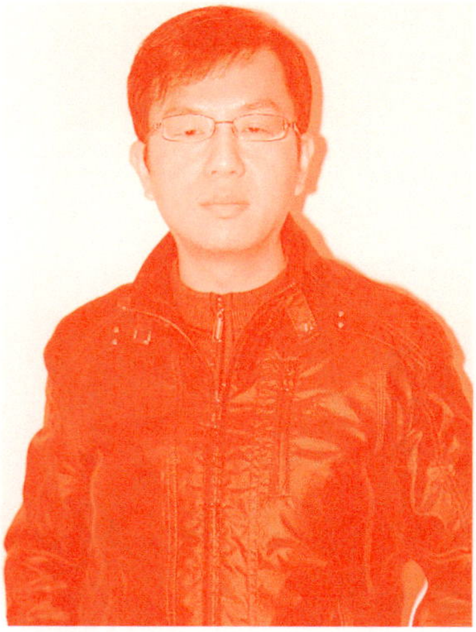
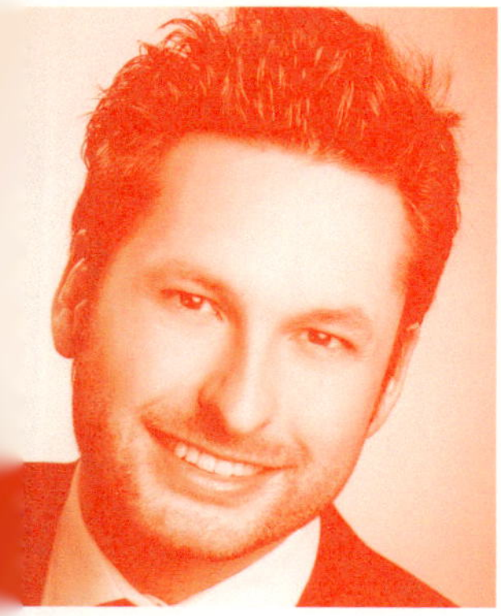
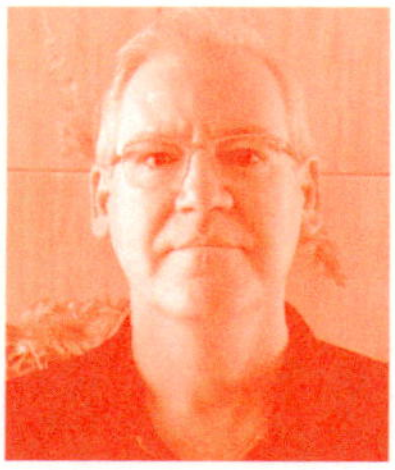

IntechOpen

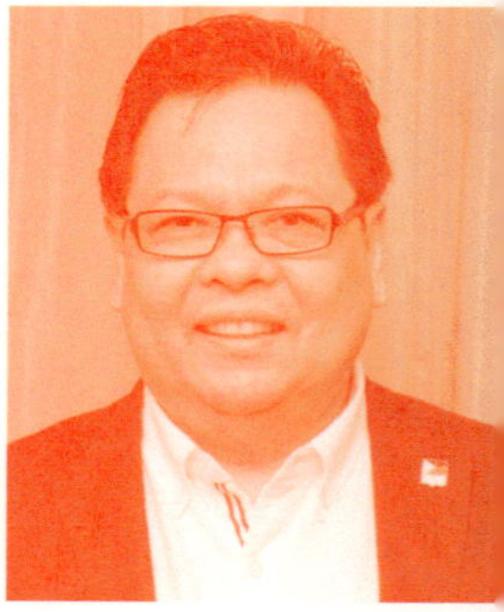
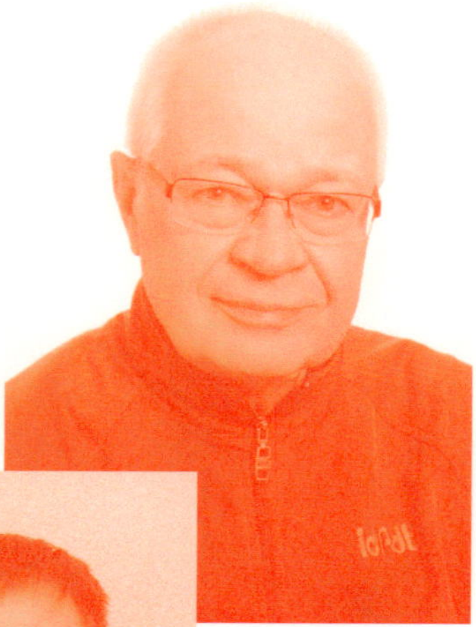
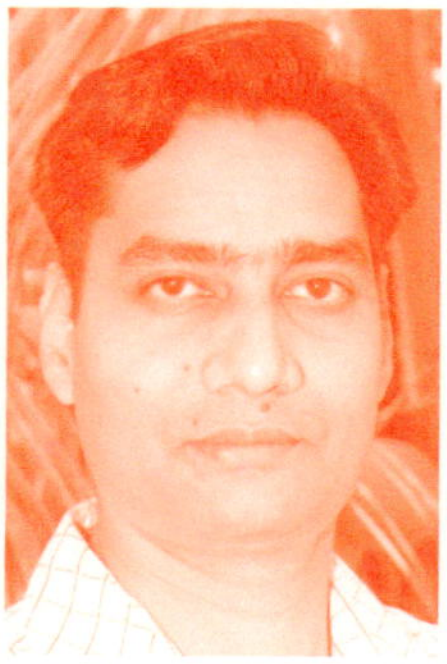
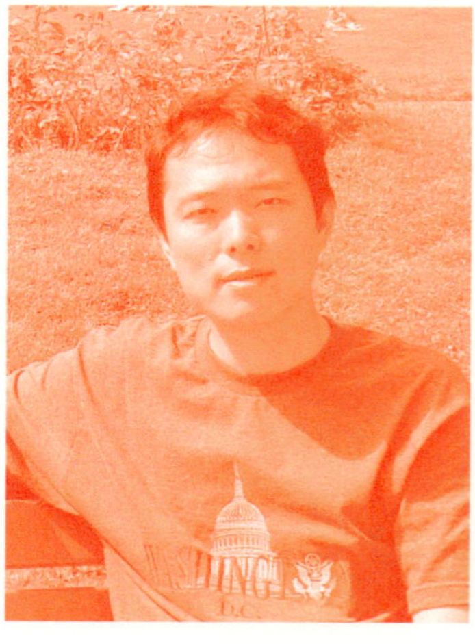
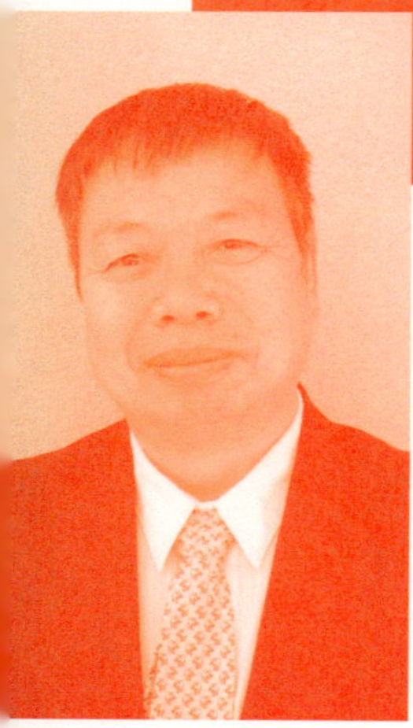
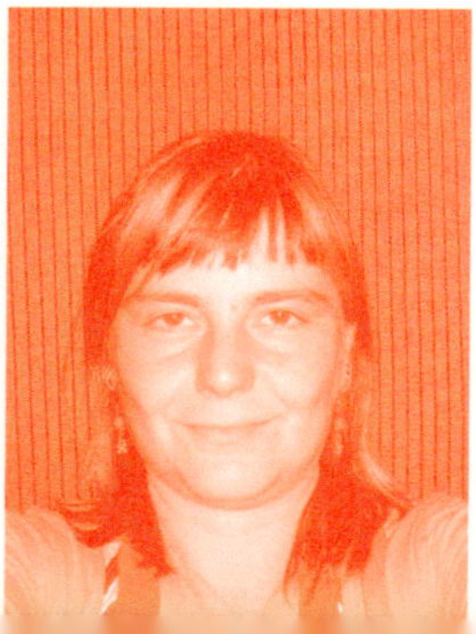

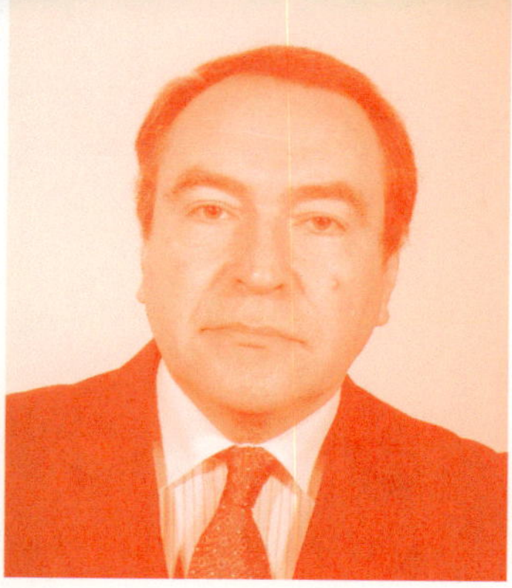
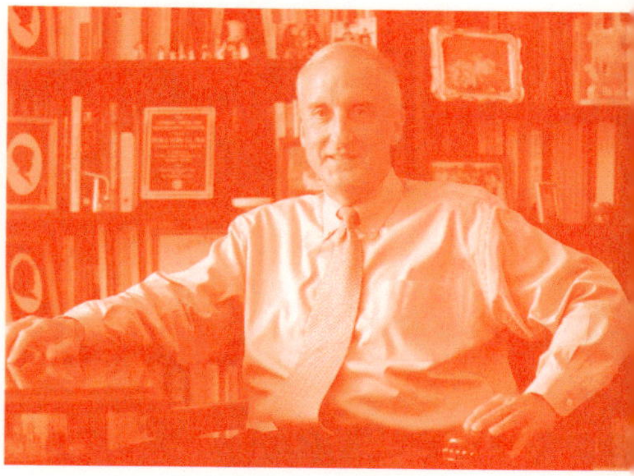
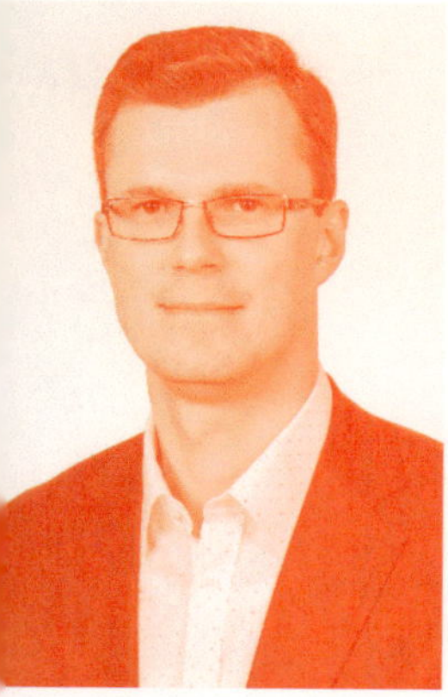
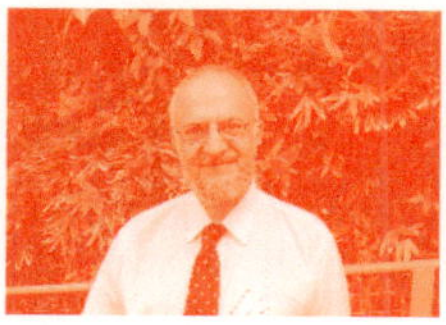
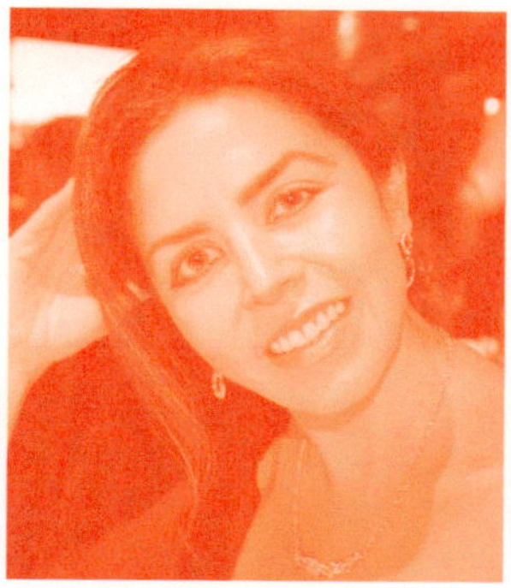

Supporting open minds since 2005

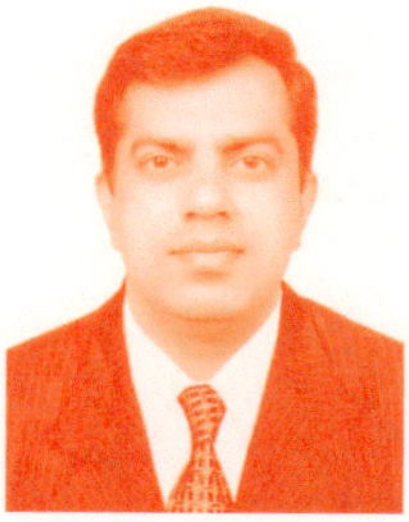
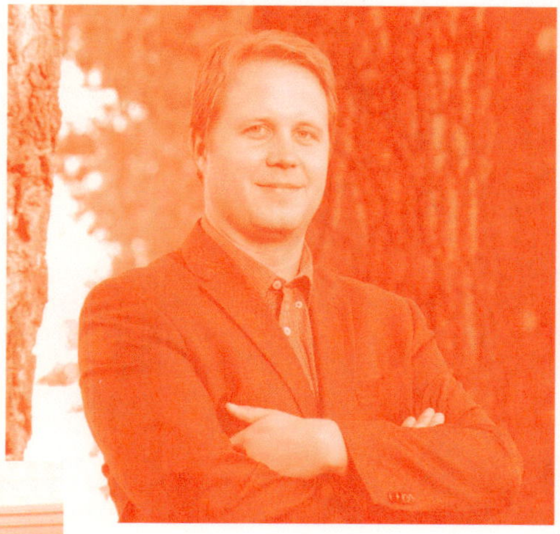
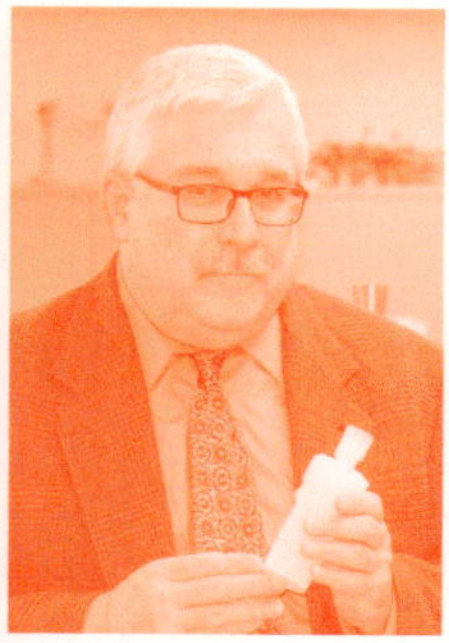
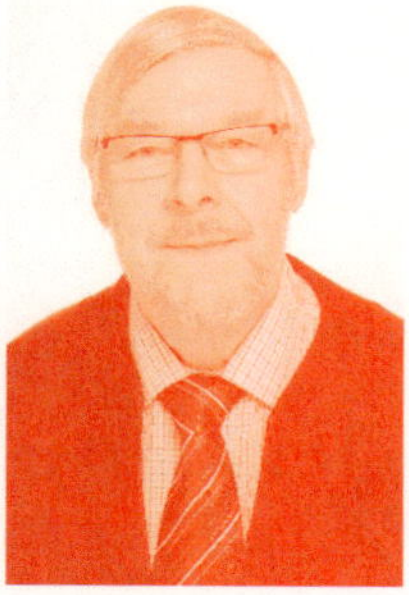
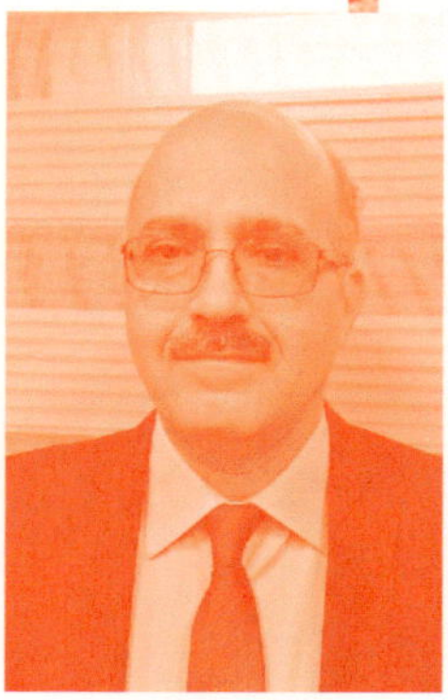
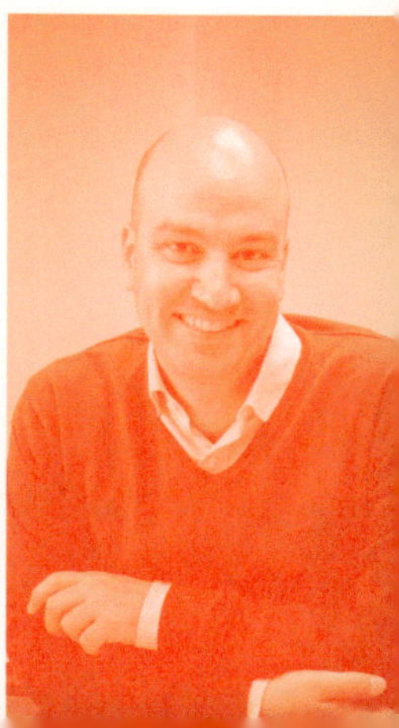
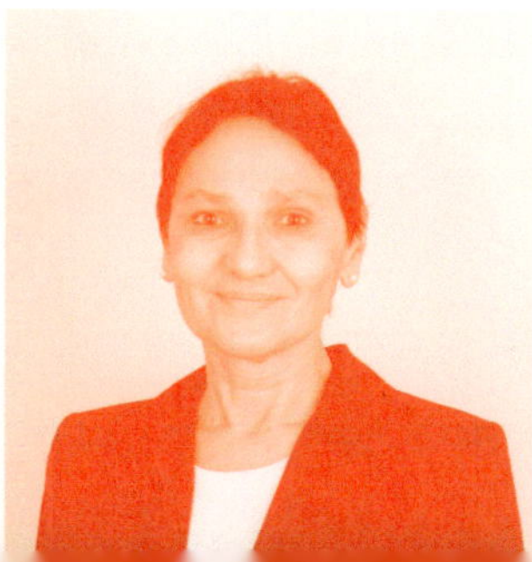

Current Trends in Cancer Management
http://dx.doi.org/10.5772/intechopen.73816
Edited by Liliana Streba, Dan Ionut Gheonea and Michael Schenker

Contributors
Mehmet Ali Koc, Suleyman Utku Celik, Cihangir Akyol, Tracey Bradshaw, Andrea Loaiza Perez, Michelle Fillion, Hülya Yazici, Aida Karachi, Saleh Alhewairini, Farmanur Rahman Khan, Richard Konichi-Dias

First published in London, United Kingdom, 2019 by IntechOpen
IntechOpen is the global imprint of INTECHOPEN LIMITED, registered in England and Wales, registration number: 11086078, The Shard, 25th floor, 32 London Bridge Street
London, SE19SG – United Kingdom
Printed in Croatia

British Library Cataloguing-in-Publication Data
A catalogue record for this book is available from the British Library

Additional hard and PDF copies can be obtained from orders@intechopen.com

Current Trends in Cancer Management
Edited by Liliana Streba, Dan Ionut Gheonea and Michael Schenker

p. cm.
Print ISBN 978-1-83880-005-5
Online ISBN 978-1-83880-006-2
eBook (PDF) ISBN 978-1-83962-207-6

For EU product safety concerns:
IN TECH d.o.o., Prolaz Marije Krucifikse Kozulić 3, 51000 Rijeka, Croatia, info@intechopen.com or visit our website at intechopen.com.

Meet the editors

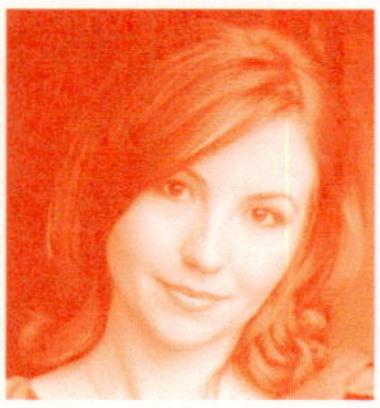

Liliana Streba, MD, PhD, Teaching Assistant at the University of Medicine and Pharmacy of Craiova, is a member of the Research Center of Gastroenterology and Hepatology of Craiova, as well as the Research Center for Microscopic Morphology and Immunology, within the same university. Her research focus is on gastric malignancies and advanced diagnostic and therapeutic techniques, having a double specialty in internal medicine and medical oncology. She has gained significant experience in pathology and microscopic diagnosis through doctoral studies and postdoctoral research activities. She has coauthored several book chapters on innovative endoscopic techniques and all significant research articles revolve around digestive cancer diagnosis and management.

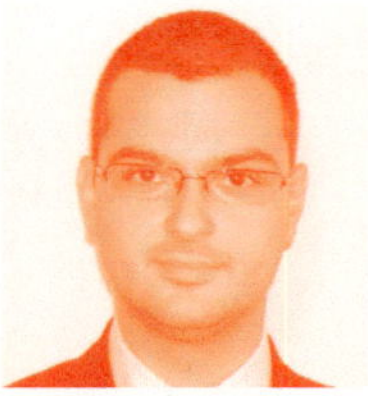

Dan Ionut Gheonea, MD, PhD, MSc, Professor at the University of Medicine and Pharmacy of Craiova and active member of the Research Center of Gastroenterology and Hepatology of Craiova (www.umfcv.ro/ccgh), is involved in the development of most of the laboratories and new techniques implemented at the university. He initiated and participated in the writing of more than 30 grant proposals. As team leader of the Elastography and Virtual Intelligence Laboratory, he developed these techniques at a national level, being invited many times as an expert to lecture on national specific meetings. He has published and communicated more than 100 papers in Romania and abroad, several of them in high-impact publications.

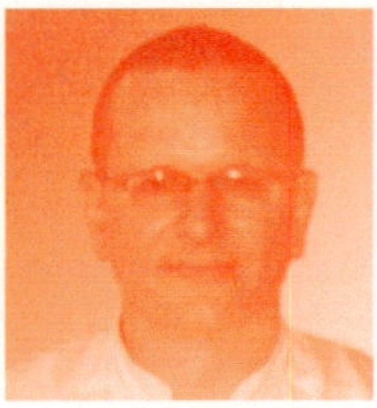

Michael Schenker, MD PhD, Lecturer at the University of Medicine and Pharmacy of Craiova, has a vast experience in conducting and promoting oncological research. He has participated in numerous research projects as team coordinator in oncology and published results in high-impact journals. His involvement in multiple large-scale multicenter trials has resulted in presented abstracts at all major oncology scientific meetings worldwide. His research interests are oncological treatment, novel therapeutic methods, and recent advancements in cancer diagnosis and management.

Contents

Preface

An early diagnosis, doubled by a comprehensive check-up and a correct choice of treatment, followed by an appropriate follow-up schedule, currently set apart successful management from failure when it comes to dealing with cancer. Although the development of new molecules constantly opens potential pathways to managing malignancies, the overall incidence and mortality rates continue to rise worldwide.

It is important to acknowledge the shifting tendencies, emerging endemic areas, and new at-risk populations in today's rapidly evolving societies. From constant exposure to stress, poor dietary and lifestyle choices, and exposure to new and more insidious polluting factors, many new challenges continue to influence the potential benefits of novel therapies. A precarious balance governs modern oncology, with the patient in the middle of this "silent war" constantly fought by medical professionals, assisted by novel tools provided by researchers from all areas of science.

Novel surgical methods, robotic procedures, and minimally invasive techniques based on newly developed devices will minimize the risk of patients, along with decreased hospitalization times, fewer consumed resources, and better economic impact. After-treatment reintegration of patients will significantly influence the global economy in the long term.

The impact of chemotherapy is further potentiated by novel lines of biological, hormonal, immunotherapeutic, and targeted medications. A more personalized type of approach is supported by recent discoveries in the fields of genetics and molecular biology.

The potential of bioinformatics, with the aid of large-scale data analysis, artificial intelligence, and similar computer-assisted tools, will become increasingly significant in the coming years.

Cancer awareness is important; the rigors of regular check-ups, starting with primary medicine and continuing in specialized centers, are the cornerstones of success stories. The successful collaboration between the poles of excellence in cancer diagnostics that exist in each country and region, their integration with primary and secondary centers, as well as the strong link with the academic world and industry researchers, will unquestionably represent the vector of success against cancer.

All these aspects require constant attention from the academic world, and the collection of interesting and diverse chapters presented within this volume will hopefully raise awareness towards interesting and novel topics. Information is being delivered faster than ever towards both medical professionals and the general population. We feel that the field of oncology is ever-changing, with major breakthroughs always waiting around the corner.

Liliana Streba and Michael Schenker
Department of Medical Oncology,
University of Medicine and Pharmacy of Craiova,
Romania

Dan Ionuț Gheonea
Department of Gastroenterology,
University of Medicine and Pharmacy of Craiova,
Romania

Section 1

Novel Approaches to Cancer Management

Chapter 1

Zebrafish (*Danio rerio*) as a Model Organism

Farmanur Rahman Khan and Saleh Sulaiman Alhewairini

Abstract

Animals as model organisms, the silent sentinels, stand watch over the environmental health of the world. These are non-human animal species which can be used to understand specific biological processes and to obtain informations which can provide an insight into working of other organisms. Among the model organisms, the zebrafish (*Danio rerio*) is one of the best leading models to study developmental biology, cancer, toxicology, drug discovery, and molecular genetics. In addition, the zebrafish is increasingly used as a genetic model organism for aquaculture species and in toxicogenomics and also to generate zebrafish disease models for application in human biomedicines. This tiny fish is a versatile model organism for many fields of research because of its easy maintenance, breeding, and transparent body during early development.

Keywords: model organisms, zebrafish, biological process, developmental biology, cancer, toxicology, drug discovery

1. Introduction

Zebrafish (*Danio rerio*) is a prominent model organism in biological researches in recent times. Zebrafish is a tropical freshwater fish, inhabitant of rivers (Ganges mainly) of Himalayan region of South Asia especially India, Nepal, Bhutan, Pakistan, Bangladesh, and Myanmar. It is a bony fish (teleost) that belongs to the family Cyprinidae under the class Actinopterygii (ray-finned fishes).

Zebrafish was first used as a biological model by George Streisinger (University of Oregon) in the 1970s because it was simpler over mouse and easy to manipulate genetically. Streisinger's colleagues especially Chuck Kimmel in his university got much impressed by the idea of using zebrafish embryo more attractive to study the development of nervous system.

The use of zebrafish as a model organism got impetus from the 1990s when it was used to develop two large genetic mutants, one by Nobel Prize winner Christiane Nusslein-Volhard in Tubingen, Germany, and the other by Wolfgang Driever and Mark Fishman in Boston, USA. The identification of mutants is one of the most important strategies for the study in various areas of biology.

Zebrafish has a lot of physiological and genetic similarities with humans, including the brain, digestive tract, musculature, vasculature, and innate immune system [1–7]. Also 70% of human disease genes have functional similarities with those of zebrafish [8].

1.1 Salient features of zebrafish as a model organism

D. Rario is preferred by scientists because of its variety of features that make it useful as a model organism. The embryo develops rapidly outside mother and optically clear and thus, easily accessible for experimentation and observation. The embryo develops very fast, and the blastula stage lasts only for 3 h, while gastrulation gets completed in 5 h; in an embryo that is about 18 h old, very well developed ears, eyes, segmenting muscles, and brain can be viewed as the embryo is transparent. By 24 h, segmentation gets completed, and most primary organ systems are formed. By 72 h, the embryo hatches out from the eggshell and within the next 2 days starts hunting for food. In a period of just 4 days, the embryo converts rapidly into a small version of adult. The rapid development simplifies development and genetic studies.

The adult zebrafish attains sexual maturity very quickly, having generation time of about 10 weeks, and also this tiny fish has good fecundity rate. When kept under optimal conditions, the zebrafish can lay about 200 eggs per week [9, 10]. Under laboratory conditions the zebrafish can spawn throughout the year that ensures the constant supply of offspring from designated pairs that makes this transparent fish a quintessential choice for large-scale genetic approaches to identify novel genes and to discover their specific functions in vertebrates [11]. The zebrafish is a very hard fish and is very easy to raise.

In addition to the features of zebrafish mentioned above, it requires very low space and maintenance cost. These features make this fish an attractive model organism for developmental, toxicological, and transgenic studies [12].

In this chapter author summarizes some of the recent advances in the area of zebrafish research, viz., developmental biology, toxicology, transgenic studies, human disease, drug discovery, cancer, etc. This review is by no means a comprehensive one but an attempt to provide a flavor to the readers some recent advances about this wonderful creature to use in potential researches.

2. Use of zebrafish in developmental biology

Much of the pioneer works that established zebrafish as a model organism were done by George Streisinger, Charles Kimmel, and their colleagues [13]. The team of these researchers studied the embryonic axis, cell lineage analysis, embryonic formation, development of central and peripheral nervous systems, muscle development, differential regulation of gene expression, etc. [14–16].

Many of the critical pathways that control development in vertebrates are highly conserved between human and zebrafish. The zebrafish genome shares a lot of similarities with human genome. About 70% of genes associated with disease in humans have functional homologs in zebrafish [8]. Realizing the importance of zebrafish model, Grunwald and Eisen used this developmental model to study the segmental structure of the brain and characterized neurons in zebrafish for the first time in a vertebrate model [17]. Nüsslein-Volhard recognized the importance of zebrafish as a vertebrate model to study developmental biology by identifying developmentally important genes [18]. The zebrafish model has been used to see the development of various systems/processes as follows.

2.1 Development of the enteric nervous system

Recently advances have been made to study the development of the enteric nervous system (ENS) using the zebrafish model. Like other vertebrates, the zebrafish gastrointestinal tract is a complex organ composed of multiple cell types like epithelial, muscular, vascular, neural, and immune cells. The gut of the zebrafish (teleost) and amniotes have structural similarities, but in teleost it is less complex as compared to amniotes [19]. The zebrafish GI tract has no distinct stomach but an enlarged area of the anterior intestine that is known as the intestinal bulb. This intestinal bulb displays patterns of motility as well as goblet cells that produce acid and neutral mucins like the stomach of mammals [20, 21]. The gut epithelium of zebrafish is simpler than that of amniotes; it lacks crypts and is arranged in an irregular broad fold rather than forming villi [21, 22]. The genes (*sox2*, *barx1*, *gata5*, *and gata6*) which are responsible for the formation of the stomach of zebrafish also resemble with that of amniotes [23].

Like that of all vertebrates, the enteric nervous system of zebrafish is also derived from neural crest [24], but it differs potentially from amniotes wherein the enteric nervous system is derived from both the vagal and sacral crests, while in the case of zebrafish, it is derived from the vagal crest only [25–28]. Enteric neural crest cell (ENCC) migration along the gut in zebrafish is also similar with that in amniotes. It takes place in two parallel chains along the length of the developing gut [25, 27, 28]. Afterward the precursors of the ENS voyage circumferentially around the gut and differentiate into the enteric neuron and glia. The final organization of the zebrafish ENS is also very simple as compared to that of amniotes; it is composed of single neuron or small group of neurons rather than more complex ganglionated myenteric and submucosal plexuses [27, 29].

2.2 Angiogenesis

Zebrafish model also has been used in the study of angiogenesis and regeneration. Angiogenesis is the process through which new blood vessels originate from preexisting vascular structures which play essential role in healthy physiological and pathological conditions. It is achieved through interaction between endothelial cells and their niche. Inadequate maintenance leads to the development of many disorders like tissue ischemia, inflammatory disorders, retinopathies, excessive vascular growth, or abnormal remodeling that promotes cancer [30].

Being a transparent vertebrate, the zebrafish has emerged as a convenient alternative to study the early development of the cardiovascular system and observe the flow of blood [31]. In zebrafish larvae the vessels and blood flow can easily be visualized by using simple dissecting microscope and also by using fluorescent proteins; the development of the blood vascular system could be examined in great details. By using confocal microscopy and time-lapse imaging, the detailed morphogenetic movements and cell shape changes can be carried out in live specimens [31].

Vascular anatomy development of zebrafish using molecular tracers during early embryonic stages has high level of similarities with other vertebrates [1, 32, 33]. In one of the experiments, the injected fluorescent microsphere was detected when lumenization and anastomosis of the vascular network were complete [34]. The same approach was adopted to compare the development of blood and lymphatic vasculatures in zebrafish [35]. The individual cell growth during vascular development also can be tracked.

For vascular development and growth, angiogenesis plays a very important role. During embryonic development, the intersegmental vessels are formed by angiogenic sprouting from the dorsal aorta, and they have been the target of studies using genetic perturbations or drugs [36]. It has been reported that mammalian malignant cells can be xenotransplanted into zebrafish embryos, and they can form tumors [37], and thus models for tumor angiogenesis have been developed [38].

2.3 Regeneration

The zebrafish exhibits remarkable capacity of regeneration even in adult stages. The caudal fin especially provides an ideal tissue for vascular regeneration studies due to its simple and fine architecture and relative transparency [39]. After successive amputations the full regeneration of the caudal fin used to take place within couple of weeks [40]. The regenerating vessels in the regenerating caudal fin originate from vein-derived cells that have angiogenic potential [41]. These cells migrate individually or in groups and assemble into the vessel in response to chemokine signaling [42].

The zebrafish as an alternative model for angiogenesis and regeneration studies provides the relevance of in vivo assays with simplicity and versatility of in vitro assays. In larvae, access to developing vasculature through fluorophore-tagged strains and small size of zebrafish makes the use of high-throughput strategies possible. In adults, the caudal fin is equally convenient as a model tissue as regenerating vessels can be observed at all stages, and the animals (zebrafish) are suitable for experimental drug manipulations [31].

3. Zebrafish as a cancer model system

Cancer is a cursed reality for millions of humans worldwide and in fact for all vertebrates. The invertebrates such as flies and nematodes also can develop anomalies in cell proliferation. Clinically and pathologically this dreaded disease is present almost exclusively in all vertebrates, from fish to humans. To understand better the formation, growth, and spread of malignant tumors, vertebrate models are imperative. Being a vertebrate the zebrafish is an ideal model to study cancer, though humans and fishes are separated from their common ancestry but biology of the cancer in both groups of organisms is the same [43]. Because of the variety of benefits to use zebrafish as a model organism which are mentioned in "Introduction," the zebrafish is adroitly exploited to carcinogenic treatment, transplantation of mammalian tumor cells, and transgenic regulations [44].

3.1 Zebrafish as a model for carcinogen effects and development of cancer studies

Fishes are exposed to many waterborne carcinogens in the wild that lead to the development of a variety of benign and malignant tumors in teleosts, and these tumors have similar histology as in humans [45, 46]. As like humans, cancer is a genetic disease in fishes as shown by melanomas which develop in *Xiphophorus* hybrids [47]. Choosing zebrafish for modeling cancer studies has many advantages. Highly conserved cancer pathways can be screened genetically using zebrafish. Primarily cancer is a disease of adults, but through mutagenesis screens, cell cycle phenotype could be examined in rapidly developing transparent embryos of the zebrafish. The genes regulating cell cycle, cell proliferation, and apoptosis have already been screened in yeast, *Drosophila* and *C. elegans*, in the similar way gene functions for these biological pathways can be screened in zebrafish to understand the events that lead to the development of cancer in any vertebrate species [43].

By inducing different gene mutations or stimulating signaling pathways through chemicals, the tumors can be induced in different organs of the zebrafish like the pancreas, liver, GI tract, vasculature, muscles, skin, and testes [46, 48–51]. It is possible to identify the interacting oncogenes via suppressor and enhancer screens which cause the formation of specific type of tumor. The mammalian tumor cells can be transplanted into the zebrafish, dispensing a novel way to study the interactions between transplanted tumor cell and vasculature of host.

3.2 Tumorigenesis

Tumorigenesis is a multistep process induced by chemical carcinogen [52], with accumulation of both epigenetic aberrations and mutations in regulatory regions of genes and disorder of signaling pathways [53, 54]. Methylation of DNA at CpG dinucleotides is an important component of epigenetic gene expression regulation [55] that causes the modulation of protein-DNA interactions [56, 57]. Aberrant methylation of CpG islands (CGT) takes place in the exonic and promoter regions [58, 59] and changes in gene expression associated with tumorigenesis. Hypermethylation of tumorigenetic genes has negative impact (regulation) over tumor suppressor genes (TSGs), DNA repair genes, and antiangiogenic genes, and it is a common quality of neoplastic cells [55, 60–63].

A variety of fishes have been used as model to study tumors induced by environmental carcinogens. Among all the zebrafish proved best for investigating embryogenesis, organogenesis, and impact of environmental carcinogen for the development of cancer [64]. Chemically induced tumors in zebrafish and humans are histopathologically similar [43, 65], and orthologous oncogenes and tumor suppressor genes (TSGs) have been identified in fishes and humans [65]. Hepatic gene expression in humans and zebrafish has revealed conservation of gene expression profiles at different stages of tumor aggressiveness between these two phylogenetically distant species [66, 67].

3.3 Xenotransplantation

Xenotransplantation represents another novel way to induce tumor in zebrafish. The most important feature of xenotransplantation is that tumor cells can be stained/marked by fluorescent stain that distinguishes transplanted cells from normal cells and helps in clear observation of developmental process of the tumor [68]. Several other types of tumor, such as pancreatic cancer, lung cancer, ovarian carcinoma, breast cancer, prostate cancer, retinoblastoma, leukemia, etc., have also been transplanted in the zebrafish [7].

3.4 Angiogenesis

Angiogenesis is the most important factor in tumor growth and subsequent metastasis. The importance of angiogenesis has been discussed well in the previous section on development. The vascular network is helpful to transport oxygen and nutrients to the cells; likewise tumor cells also get the supply of all these materials. Because of this reason, the development and the capability of the formation of blood vessels within the tumor determine the malignancy of the cancer as well as influence the therapeutic effects and prognosis. The endothelial cells of the vascular system can be stained by fluorescent dye/protein that helps to visualize the neovascularization of tiny tumor at the earliest stage, and metastasizing tumor cells can be tracked explicitly at cellular level [7]. The vascular system of tumor has always been the target of antitumor therapies; it is evident from research and clinical observations that if angiogenesis inhibitors are used in combination with chemotherapy, it can improve the outcome in cancer patients [69].

3.5 Skin cancer

Skin or dermal cancers represent the most common type of cutaneous malignancy globally, which includes melanoma and carcinoma of squamous cells [70]. Melanoma is the most pernicious form of skin cancer among all types of skin cancers and has mortality rate over 80% [71, 72]. Melanoma usually develops in the pigmented epidermal cells (melanocytes), which are responsible for the production of melanin. In the beginning of melanoma, it is restricted to the epidermis because of the radial growth phase (RGP) of melanoma, and it can be removed by surgical excision [73]. In later stages of tumor progression, the melanoma cells invade the subcutaneous tissues due to vertical growth phase (VGP) of melanoma and eventually lead toward the metastatic phase. At this stage, very limited therapeutic options are available, and melanoma frequently deteriorates and becomes untreatable [73, 74].

Cutaneous squamous cell carcinoma (cSCC) mostly develops due to UV radiation exposure of epidermal cells, namely, keratinocytes, in which uncontrolled proliferation starts [75]. cSCC accounts for the most frequent type of non-melanoma cutaneous cancer and constitutes about 20% of all skin malignancies [75, 76].

SCCs are curable in situ by surgical excision. Metastatic SCCs are responsible for majority of deaths due to non-melanoma skin cancer [70]. Head and neck squamous cell carcinoma (HNSCC) develops in various places such as the oropharynx and laryngopharynx which is very common worldwide [77]. Especially oral squamous cell carcinoma (OSCC) accounts for about 24% of HNSCC with a mortality rate of 2 million deaths every year [76, 78].

Zebrafish is a powerful in vivo tool to study pathologies and treatment for skin cancer (melanoma and SCC). The zebrafish can be used to study melanoma development, progression, drug screening, and treatment. The zebrafish model has been exploited recently to recognize the key molecules which are responsible for the development of cutaneous squamous cell carcinoma (cSCC) and head and neck squamous cell carcinoma (HNSCC) [72] as well as for SCC target therapies [79].

3.6 Tumor metastasis

Metastasis is a multistep and complex process in which tumor cells penetrate in the vascular system and spread deep in parenchymatous tissues [80]. For better therapeutic practices like development of antitumor drugs and advancements of clinical treatments, the insight into mechanism of tumor metastasis is very helpful. Because of many significant disadvantages in the previous studies using in vivo mouse model, the metastasis process cannot be abstracted properly, but zebrafish cancer model has overcome the drawback of previous models and has shown exceptional strengths. The adaptive immune system in larvae of zebrafish usually develops after 14 DPF, which provides very conducive environment for survival of transplanted cancer cells and metastasis [81], and the process of tumor metastasis can be observed through the transparent body of zebrafish under microscope. To better understand the process of metastasis, the transplanted tumor cells can be stained/treated by dye like CM-Dil or may be labeled by red fluorescent protein (RFP) [82]. Mammalian tumor cells treated with red fluorescent protein when injected into transgenic zebrafish, the process of tumor cell metastasis and angiogenesis can be viewed well after 48 h of transplantation [83]. By using zebrafish, the suppressing or promoting factors for metastasis can be identified. In RFP treated U87 glioma stem cells (GSCs), when transplanted into the yolk sac of the zebrafish embryo, the various invasive stages of GSCs like approaching, cluster formation, invasion, migration, and transmigration can be observed clearly at 48 h postinjection [83].

4. Toxicology and drug discovery

As discussed previously in Section 1, because of many advantages, the zebrafish has recently emerged as a prominent model for toxicological studies and drug discovery. The effects of drugs on growth and development can be examined visually through length and shape of the zebrafish body as well as the morphology of internal organs such as the brain, liver, cardiovascular system, pancreas, intestine, kidney, notochord, etc. The zebrafish model also has been used to know the organ function assays and assessment of drug effect [84].

Zebrafish embryos are used as predictive model to assess the toxicity in mammals. The lethal concentration (LC_{50}) of different chemicals has been determined in embryos of zebrafish and has been compared with the mammalian LC_{50}, and it has been found that median lethal dose of zebrafish is lower than mammals [84]. The effects of drugs on specific organs have also been studied, and it has been found that organ toxicity is similar in both zebrafish and mammals. The drugs that were used to evaluate the organ toxicity were gentamicin, cisplatin, vinblastine, quinine, neomycin, doxorubicin, dexamethasone, cyclosporin A, caffeine, camptothecin, MPA, fluorouracil, etc. [85–90].

4.1 Drug toxicity

In drug development, the toxicity plays a major role. Due to the toxicity problem, many new drugs have been declined by the FDA. The evaluation of toxicity of drug is very essential to know the end points of toxicity, dose-response relationships, and mechanism of toxicity and also to determine the toxicodynamics of the drug [91].

The zebrafish is acquiring the reputation rapidly as a promising model animal to study drug and chemical toxicology [92, 93]. The toxicity of some of the important drugs has been examined using the zebrafish model, for instance, Amanuma et al. [94] developed a test in which susceptible zebrafish was used to detect small molecule-induced mutagenesis. The embryos of zebrafish were utilized to compare the developmental toxicity resulting from the exposure to ethanol or acetaldehyde [95]. Toxicity of antirheumatic drug like diclofenac was evaluated by using zebrafish. Now, zebrafish has got the status of a successful animal model to study drug toxicity and toxicology caused by environmental contaminants [91].

4.2 Zebrafish and drug discovery

The zebrafish model has been used potentially in drug discovery and to know the effects of neurotoxic, ototoxic, and neuroprotectant drugs. The process of drug discovery is divided into four main components: screening of lead compounds, target identification, target validation, and assay development [96]. The process of target identification involves the recognition of target gene or protein which when modulated by a drug can have positive effects on the progression of disease. After identification of possible target, the validation process of target begins through determination of protein function and assessment of the druggability of the target [84, 97–99]. Zebrafish has great role in each of these areas of drug discovery.

4.3 Angiogenesis

The angiogenesis has already been discussed earlier in detail in previous sections on development and cancer. The impact of various proangiogenic compounds like simvastatine or penicillamine[20] or antiangiogenic compounds like vandetanib or PTK787 can be assessed well and visualized through the development of the vascular system in transparent zebrafish embryo [84].

4.4 Cardiotoxicity

In drug development, cardiotoxicity is one of the major concerns. Through the transparent zebrafish embryo, various cardiac functions like heart rate, rhythm, contraction, circulation, etc. can be assessed directly. It has been demonstrated well that toxic effects of ten cardiotoxic agents in zebrafish embryos have similar impact as in humans [100]. Treatment with terfenadine and clomipramine caused severe impairment of cardiac functions, edema, hemorrhage, arrested heartbeat, and even death. These results in zebrafish exhibit similarities with humans [101]. Another group of researchers proposed to use a transgenic model for high-throughput testing of small molecules that modulate the heart rate of the zebrafish embryo [102]. Thus, zebrafish is a suitable model for preliminary screening of molecules which have potential therapeutic or toxic effects.

5. Human disease and zebrafish

Most of the tissues and organs found in humans and zebrafish are the same except lungs and prostrate and mammary glands. The cloning of mutated genes screened for specific phenotypes in zebrafish has similarities in humans and thus serves as model for human disease and to study underlying mechanisms. The first human disease identified using zebrafish was a blood disorder involving specific defect in hemoglobin production through ALAS2 mutated gene [103].

Many other mutants which show phenotypic similarities to human disease have been screened and identified. These include neurological disorders [104], hematological disorder [105, 106], cardiovascular diseases [107], muscle disease [108] and cancers [109, 110], Parkinson's disease [111], anxiety, and posttraumatic stress disorder [112].

6. Zebrafish as a model organism for aquaculture species

Among different fish species of interest to aquaculture, zebrafish is genetically more tractable. The zebrafish model is used commercially in many areas of aquaculture such as in the identification of genes involved in the development of the muscles, bones, and fats, the metabolism of nutrients, disease, and stress pathways and also behavioral traits. The drugs which affect the physiology of the fishes can be tested easily in zebrafish especially their effect on a range of alleles to assess their genetic property [113]. Many researches have been done regarding the improvement of diet and their husbandry to improve the growth rate and reduce stress and disease in many fish species like gilthead seabream, seabass, rainbow trout, Atlantic salmon, tilapia, catfish, cod, etc. [10]. The zebrafish disease models are being used in various infections of aquaculture, for instance, tuberculosis and streptococcal and salmonella infections [114].

7. Conclusion

Zebrafish is a successful and versatile animal model system, offering a tool to model gene function, development of various organ systems, cancer studies, toxicology, drug discovery, human disease and disorders and also in aquaculture, etc. because low cost and easy maintenance, transparent embryo, easy manipulation, high fecundity, and rapid embryonic development favor the zebrafish as an attractive model for in vivo assays with simplicity and versatility of in vitro assays over mammalian models which lack all of these benefits. The future of zebrafish as model organism is very bright. In coming years, an increased number of reports are expected on the application of zebrafish as an effective bioindicator.

Conflict of interest

The author declares that there is no conflict of interest.

Author details

Farmanur Rahman Khan[1*] and Saleh Sulaiman Alhewairini[2]

1 Department of Biology, Deanship of Educational Services, Qassim University, Al Qassim, Buraidah, Saudi Arabia

2 Department of Plant Production and Protection, College of Agriculture and Veterinary Medicine, Qassim University, Al Qassim, Buraidah, Saudi Arabia

*Address all correspondence to: insectqh11@gmail.com

References

[1] Gore AV, Monzo K, Cha YR, Pan W, Weinstein BM. Vascular development in the zebrafish. Cold Spring Harbor Perspectives in Medicine. 2012;**2**(5):a006684

[2] Kanungo J, Cuevas E, Ali SF, Paule MG. Zebrafish model in drug safety assessment. Current Pharmaceutical Design. 2014;**20**(34):5416-5429

[3] Kalueff AV, Stewart AM, Gerlai R. Zebrafish as an emerging model for studying complex brain disorders. Trends in Pharmacological Sciences. 2014;**35**(2):63-75

[4] Guyon JR, Steffen LS, Howell MH, Pusack TJ, Lawrence C, Kunkel LM. Modeling human muscle disease in zebrafish. Biochimica et Biophysica Acta. 2007;**1772**(2):205-215

[5] Weinstein B. Vascular cell biology in vivo: A new piscine paradigm? Trends in Cell Biology. 2002;**12**(9):439-445

[6] Lieschke GJ, Oates AC, Crowhurst MO, Ward AC, Layton JE. Morphologic and functional characterization of granulocytes and macrophages in embryonic and adult zebrafish. Blood. 2001;**98**(10):3087-3096

[7] Zhao S, Huang J, Ye J. A fresh look at zebrafish from the perspective of cancer research. Journal of Experimental & Clinical Cancer Research. 2015;**34**:80. DOI: 10.1186/s13046-015-0196-8

[8] Santoriello C, Zon LI. Hooked! Modeling human disease in zebrafish. The Journal of Clinical Investigation. 2012;**122**(7):2337-2343

[9] Brand M, Granato M, Nusslein-Volhard C. Keeping and raising zebrafish. In: Nusslein-Volhard C, Dahm R, editors. Zebrafish: A Practical Approach. Oxford: Oxford University Press; 2002. pp. 7-37

[10] Carpio Y, Estrada MP. Zebrafish as a genetic model organism. Biotecnologia Aplicada. 2006;**23**:265-270

[11] Pelegri F. Mutagenesis. In: Nusslein-Volhard C, Dahm R, editors. Zebrafish: A Practical Approach. Oxford: Oxford University Press; 2002. pp. 145-174

[12] Lele Z, Krone PH. The zebrafish as a model system in developmental, toxicological and transgenic research. Biotechnology Advances. 1996;**14**(1):57-72

[13] Kimmel CB. Genetics and early development of zebrafish. Trends in Genetics. 1989;**5**:283-288

[14] Chakrabarti S, Streisinger G, Singer F, Walker C. Frequency of gamma-ray induced specific locus and recessive lethal mutations in mature germ cells of the zebrafish, *Brachydanio rerio*. Genetics. 1983;**103**:109-123

[15] Streisinger G, Singer F, Walker C, Knauber D, Dower N. Segregation analyses and gene-centromere distances in zebrafish. Genetics. 1986;**112**:311-319

[16] Walker C, Streisinger G. Induction of mutations by gamma-rays in pregonial germ cells of zebrafish embryos. Genetics. 1983;**103**:125-136

[17] Grunwald DJ, Eisen JS. Headwaters of the zebrafish—Emergence of a new model vertebrate. Nature Reviews. Genetics. 2002;**3**:717-724

[18] Nüsslein-Volhard C, Wieschaus E. Mutations affecting segment number and polarity in Drosophila. Nature. 1980;**287**:795-801

[19] Wallace KN, Akhter S, Smith EM, Lorent K, Pack M. Intestinal growth and differentiation in zebrafish. Mechanisms of Development. 2005;**122**:157-173

[20] Holmberg A, Olsson C, Hennig GW. TTX-sensitive and TTX-insensitive control of spontaneous gut motility in the developing zebrafish (*Danio rerio*) larvae. The Journal of Experimental Biology. 2007;**210**:1084-1091

[21] Ng AN, de Jong-Curtain TA, Mawdsley DJ, White SJ, Shin J, Appel B, et al. Formation of the digestive system in zebrafish: III. Intestinal epithelium morphogenesis. Developmental Biology. 2005;**286**:114-135

[22] Wallace AS, Burns AJ. Development of the enteric nervous system, smooth muscle and interstitial cells of Cajal in the human gastrointestinal tract. Cell and Tissue Research. 2005;**319**:367-382

[23] Muncan V, Faro A, Haramis AP, Hurlstone AF, Wienholds E, van Es J, et al. T-cell factor 4 (Tcf7l2) maintains proliferative compartments in zebrafish intestine. EMBO Reports. 2007;**8**:966-973

[24] Kelsh RN, Eisen JS. The zebrafish colourless gene regulates development of non-ectomesenchymal neural crest derivatives. Development. 2000;**127**:515-525

[25] Elworthy S, Pinto JP, Pettifer A, Cancela ML, Kelsh RN. Phox2b function in the enteric nervous system is conserved in zebrafish and is sox10-dependent. Mechanisms of Development. 2005;**122**:659-669

[26] Furness JB. The Enteric Nervous System. Oxford: John Wiley and Sons Ltd.; 2006

[27] Olden T, Akhtar T, Beckman SA, Wallace KN. Differentiation of the zebrafish enteric nervous system and intestinal smooth muscle. Genesis. 2008;**46**:484-498

[28] Shepherd IT, Pietsch J, Elworthy S, Kelsh RN, Raible DW. Roles for GFRalpha1 receptors in zebrafish enteric nervous system development. Development. 2004;**131**:241-249

[29] Tiffany AH, Shepherd IT, Burns AJ. Enteric nervous system development in avian and zebrafish models. Developmental Biology. 2016;**417**(2):129-138. DOI: 10.1016/j.ydbio.2016.05.017

[30] Pandya N, Dhalla N, Santani D. Angiogenesis—A new target for future therapy. Vascular Pharmacology. 2006;**44**:265-274. DOI: 10.1016/j.vph.2006.01.005

[31] Chávez MN, Aedo G, Fierro FA, Allende ML, Egaña JT. Zebrafish as an emerging model organism to study angiogenesis in development and regeneration. Frontiers in Physiology. 2016;7:56. DOI: 10.3389/fphys.2016.00056

[32] Isogai S, Horiguchi M, Weinstein BM. The vascular anatomy of the developing zebrafish: An atlas of embryonic and early larval development. Developmental Biology. 2001;**230**:278-301. DOI: 10.1006/dbio.2000.9995

[33] Ellertsdóttir E, Lenard A, Blum Y, Krudewig A, Herwig L, Affolter M. Vascular morphogenesis in the zebrafish embryo. Developmental Biology. 2001;**341**:56-65. DOI: 10.1016/j.ydbio.2009.10.035

[34] Küchler AM, Gjini E, Peterson-Maduro J, Cancilla B, Wolburg H, Schulte-Merker S. Development of the zebrafish lymphatic system requires VEGFC signaling. Current Biology. 2006;**16**:1244-1248. DOI: 10.1016/j.cub.2006.05.026

[35] Coffindaffer-Wilson M, Craig MP, Hove JR. Determination of lymphatic vascular identity and developmental timecourse in zebrafish (*Danio rerio*). Lymphology. 2011;**44**:1-12

[36] Schuermann A, Helker CS, Herzog W. Angiogenesis in zebrafish. Seminars in Cell & Developmental Biology. 2014;**31**:106-114. DOI: 10.1016/j.semcdb.2014.04.037

[37] Haldi M, Ton C, Seng WL, McGrath P. Human melanoma cells transplanted into zebrafish proliferate, migrate, produce melanin, form masses and stimulate angiogenesis in zebrafish. Angiogenesis. 2006;**9**:139-151. DOI: 10.1007/s10456-006-9040-2

[38] Tobia C, De Sena G, Presta M. Zebrafish embryo, a tool to study tumor angiogenesis. The International Journal of Developmental Biology. 2011;**55**:505-509. DOI: 10.1387/ijdb.103238ct

[39] Poss KD, Keating MT, Nechiporuk A. Tales of regeneration in zebrafish. Developmental Dynamics. 2003;**226**:202-210. DOI: 10.1002/dvdy.10220

[40] Azevedo A, Grotek B, Jacinto A, Weidinger G, Saúde L, Karl M. The regenerative capacity of the zebrafish caudal fin is not affected by repeated amputations. PLoS One. 2011;**6**:e22820. DOI: 10.1371/journal.pone.0022820

[41] Xu C, Hasan SS, Schmidt I, Rocha SF, Pitulescu ME, Bussmann J. Arteries are formed by vein-derived endothelial tip cells. Nature Communications. 2014;**5**:5758. DOI: 10.1038/ncomms6758

[42] Hasan SS, Siekmann AF. The same but different: Signaling pathways in control of endothelial cell migration. Current Opinion in Cell Biology. 2015;**36**:86-92. DOI: 10.1016/j.ceb.2015.07.009

[43] Amatruda JF, Shepard JL, Stern HM, Zon LI. Zebrafish as a cancer model system. Cancer Cell. 2002;**1**:229-231

[44] Mizgirev I, Revskoy S. Generation of clonal zebrafish lines and transplantable hepatic tumors. Nature Protocols. 2010;**5**(3):383-394

[45] Hawkins WE, Overstreet RM, Fournie JW, Walker WW. Development of aquarium fish models for environmental carcinogenesis: Tumor induction in seven species. Journal of Applied Toxicology. 1985;**5**:261-264

[46] Spitsbergen JM, Tsai HW, Reddy A, Miller T, Arbogast D, Hendricks JD, et al. Neoplasia in zebrafish (*Danio rerio*) treated with 7,12-dimethylbenz[a]anthracene by two exposure routes at different developmental stages. Toxicologic Pathology. 2000;**28**:705-715

[47] Walter RB, Kazianis S. Xiphophorus interspecies hybrids as genetic models of induced neoplasia. ILAR Journal. 2001;**42**:299-321

[48] Basten SG, Davis EE, Gillis AJ, van Rooijen E, Stoop H, Babala N, et al. Mutations in LRRC50 predispose zebrafish and humans to seminomas. PLoS Genetics. 2013;**9**(4):e1003384

[49] Lam SH, Wu YL, Vega VB, Miller LD, Spitsbergen J, Tong Y, et al. Conservation of gene expression signatures between zebrafish and human liver tumors and tumor progression. Nature Biotechnology. 2006;**24**(1):73-75

[50] Mizgireuv IV, Revskoy SY. Transplantable tumor lines generated in clonal zebrafish. Cancer Research. 2006;**66**(6):3120-3125

[51] Spitsbergen JM, Tsai HW, Reddy A, Miller T, Arbogast D, Hendricks JD, et al. Neoplasia in zebrafish (*Danio rerio*) treated with N-methyl-N'-nitro-Nnitrosoguanidine by three exposure routes at different developmental stages. Toxicologic Pathology. 2000;**28**(5):716-725

[52] Counts JL, Goodman JI. Hypomethylation of DNA: A

nongenotoxic mechanism involved in tumor promotion. Toxicology Letters. 1995;**82/83**:663-672

[53] Tischoff I, Tannapfel A. DNA methylation in hepatocellular carcinoma. World Journal of Gastroenterology. 2008;**14**(11):1741-1748

[54] Gronbaek K, Hother C, Jones PA. Epigenetic changes in cancer. APMIS. 2007;**115**:1039-1059

[55] Rauch T, Wang Z, Zhang X, Zhong X, Wu X, Lau SK, et al. Homeobox gene methylation in lung cancer studied by genome-wide analysis with microarray-based methylation CpG island recovery assay. PNAS. 2007;**104**(13):5527-5532

[56] Jones PA, Takai D. The role of DNA methylation in mammalian epigenetics. Science. 2001;**293**:1068-1070

[57] Pomraning KR, Smith KM, Freitag M. Genome-wide high throughput analysis of DNA methylation in eukaryotes. Methods. 2009;**47**:142-150

[58] Weber M, Davies JJ, Wittig D, Oakeley EJ, Haase M, Lam WL, et al. Chromosome-wide and promoter-specific analyses identify sites of different DNA methylation in normal and transformed human cells. Nature Genetics. 2005;**37**(8):853-862

[59] Takai D, Jones PA. Comprehensive analysis of CpG islands in human chromosome 21 and 22. PNAS. 2002;**99**(6):3740-3745

[60] Rauch T, Li H, Wu X, Pfeifer GP. MIRA-assisted microarray analysis, a new technology for the determination of DNA methylation patterns, identifies frequent methylation of homeodomain-containing genes in lung cancer cells. Cancer Research. 2006;**66**(16):7939-7947

[61] Lopez J, Percharde M, Coley HM, Webb A, Crook T. The context and potential of epigenetics in oncology. British Journal of Cancer. 2009;**100**:571-577

[62] Momparler RL, Bovenzi V. DNA methylation and cancer. Journal of Cellular Physiology. 2000;**183**:145-154

[63] Baylin SB, Herman JG. DNA hypermethylation in tumourigenesis. Epigenetics joins genetics. Trends in Genetics. 2000;**16**(4):168-174

[64] Bailey GS, Williams DE, Hendricks JD. Fish models for environmental carcinogenesis: The rainbow trout. Environmental Health Perspectives. 1996;**104**(1):5-21

[65] Berghmans S, Jette C, Langenau D, Hsu K, Stewart R, Look T, et al. Making waves in cancer research: New models in the zebrafish. BioTechniques. 2005;**39**:227-237

[66] Larn S, Wu Y, Vega VB, Miller LD, Spitsbergen J, Tong Y, et al. Conservation of gene expression signature between zebrafish and human liver tumors and tumor progression. Nature Biotechnology. 2006;**24**(1):73-75

[67] Mirbahai L, Williams T, Zhan H, Gong Z, Chipman JK. Comprehensive profiling of zebrafish hepatic proximal promoter CpG island methylation and its modification during chemical carcinogenesis. BMC Genomics. 2011;**12**:3

[68] Smith AC, Raimondi AR, Salthouse CD, Ignatius MS, Blackburn JS, Mizgirev IV, et al. High-throughput cell transplantation establishes that tumorinitiating cells are abundant in zebrafish T-cell acute lymphoblastic leukemia. Blood. 2010;**115**(16):3296-3303

[69] Bellou S, Pentheroudakis G, Murphy C, Fotsis T. Anti-angiogenesis in cancer therapy: Hercules and hydra. Cancer Letters. 2013;**338**(2):219-228

[70] Von Massenhausen A, Sanders C, Bragelmann J, Konantz M, Queisser A, Vogel W, et al. Targeting DDR2 in head and neck squamous cell carcinoma with dasatinib. International Journal of Cancer. 2016;**139**:2359-2369

[71] Ochoa-Alvarez JA, Krishnan H, Pastorino JG, Nevel E, Kephart D, Lee JJ, et al. Antibody and lectin target podoplanin to inhibit oral squamous carcinoma cell migration and viability by distinct mechanisms. Oncotarget. 2016;**6**:9045-9060

[72] Shin YS, Cha HY, Lee BS, Kang SU, Hwang HS, Kwon HC, et al. Anti-cancer effect of luminacin, a marine microbial extract, in head and neck squamous cell carcinoma progression via autophagic cell death. Cancer Research and Treatment. 2016;**48**:738-752

[73] Michailidou C, Jones M, Walker P, Kamarashev J, Kelly A, Hurlstone AF. Dissecting the roles of Raf and PI3K-signalling pathways in melanoma formation and progression in a zebrafish model. Disease Models & Mechanisms. 2009;**2**:399-411

[74] Fernandez Del Ama L, Jones M, Walker P, Chapman A, Braun JA, Mohr J, et al. Reprofiling using a zebrafish melanoma model reveals drugs cooperating with targeted therapeutics. Oncotarget. 2016;7:40348-40361

[75] Martins VL, Caley MP, Moore K, Szentpetery Z, Marsh ST, Murrell DF, et al. Suppression of TGFβ and angiogenesis by type VII collagen in cutaneous SCC. Journal of the National Cancer Institute. 2015;**108**(1):djv293. https://doi.org/10.1093/jnci/djv293

[76] Xiong P, Xiao LY, Yang R, Guo Q, Zhao YQ, Li W, et al. Flotillin-1 promotes cell growth and metastasis in oral squamous cell carcinoma. Neoplasma. 2013;**60**:395-405

[77] Bootorabi F, Manouchehri H, Changizi R, Barker H, Palazzo E, Saltari A, et al. Zebrafish as a model organism for the development of drugs for skin cancer. International Journal of Molecular Sciences. 2017;**18**:E1550

[78] Xiong P, Li YX, Tang YT, Chen HG. Proteomic analyses of Sirt1-mediated cisplatin resistance in OSCC cell line. The Protein Journal. 2011;**30**:499-508

[79] Jung DW, Kim J, Che ZM, Oh ES, Kim G, Eom SH, et al. A triazine compound S06 inhibits proinvasive crosstalk between carcinoma cells and stromal fibroblasts via binding to heat shock protein 90. Chemistry & Biology. 2011;**18**:1581-1590

[80] Eccles SA, Welch DR. Metastasis: Recent discoveries and novel treatment strategies. Lancet. 2007;**369**(9574):1742-1757

[81] Traver D, Herbomel P, Patton EE, Murphey RD, Yoder JA, Litman GW, et al. The zebrafish as a model organism to study development of the immune system. Advances in Immunology. 2003;**81**:253-330

[82] Marques IJ, Weiss FU, Vlecken DH, Nitsche C, Bakkers J, Lagendijk AK, et al. Metastatic behaviour of primary human tumours in a zebrafish xenotransplantation model. BMC Cancer. 2009;**9**:128

[83] Yang XJ et al. A novel zebrafish xenotransplantation model for study of glioma stem cell invasion. PLoS One. 2013;**8**(4):e61801

[84] Kari G, Rodeck U, Dicker AP. Zebrafish: An emerging model system for human disease and drug discovery. Clinical Pharmacology and Therapeutics. 2007;**82**(1):70-80

[85] Zhang C, Willett C, Fremgen T. Zebrafish: An animal model for toxicological studies. Current

Protocols in Toxicology. 2003. DOI: 10.1002/0471140856.tx0107s17

[86] Daroczi B, Kari G, McAleer MF, Wolf JC, Rodeck U, Dicker AP. In vivo radioprotection by the fullerene nanoparticle DF-1 as assessed in a zebrafish model. Clinical Cancer Research. 2006;**12**:7086-7091

[87] Langheinrich U, Hennen E, Stott G, Vacun G. Zebrafish as a model organism for the identification and characterization of drugs and genes affecting p53 signaling. Current Biology. 2002;**12**:2023-2028

[88] McAleer MF et al. Novel use of zebrafish as a vertebrate model to screen radiation protectors and sensitizers. International Journal of Radiation Oncology, Biology, Physics. 2005;**61**:10-13

[89] Ton C, Parng C. The use of zebrafish for assessing ototoxic and otoprotective agents. Hearing Research. 2005;**208**:79-88

[90] Wu X, Zhong H, Song J, Damoiseaux R, Yang Z, Lin S. Mycophenolic acid is a potent inhibitor of angiogenesis. Arteriosclerosis, Thrombosis, and Vascular Biology. 2006;**26**:2414-2416

[91] Chakraborty C, Hsu CH, Wen ZH, Lin CS, Agoramoorthy G. Zebrafish: A complete animal model for in vivo drug discovery and development. Current Drug Metabolism. 2009;**10**:116-124

[92] Spitsbergen JM, Kent ML. The state of the art of the zebrafish model for toxicology and toxicologic pathology research—Advantages and current limitations. Toxicologic Pathology. 2003;**31**:62-87

[93] Rubinstein AL. Zebrafish assays for drug toxicity screening. Expert Opinion on Drug Metabolism & Toxicology. 2006;**2**(2):231-240

[94] Amanuma K, Takeda H, Amanuma H, Aoki Y. Transgenic zebrafish for detecting mutations caused by compounds in aquatic environments. Nature Biotechnology. 2000;**18**(1):62-65

[95] Reimers MJ, Flockton AR, Tanguay RL. Ethanol- and acetaldehyde-mediated developmental toxicity in zebrafish. Neurotoxicology and Teratology. 2004;**26**(6):769-781

[96] Handen JS. The industrialization of drug discovery. Drug Discovery Today. 2002;7(2):83-85

[97] Eckstein J. ISOA/ARF drug development tutorial. http://www.alzforum.org/drg/tut/tutorial.asp

[98] Lindsay MA. Target discovery. Nature Reviews. Drug Discovery. 2003;**2**(10):831-838

[99] Frank SD. Target-based drug discovery: Is something wrong? Drug Discovery Today. 2005;**10**(2):139-147

[100] Langheinrich U, Vacun G, Wagner T. Zebrafish embryos express an orthologue of HERG and are sensitive toward a range of QT-prolonging drugs inducing severe arrhythmia. Toxicology and Applied Pharmacology. 2003;**193**:370-382

[101] Lawson ND, Weinstein BM. In vivo imaging of embryonic vascular development using transgenic zebrafish. Developmental Biology. 2002;**248**:307-318

[102] Burns CG, Milan DJ, Grande EJ, Rottbauer W, MacRae CA, Fishman MC. High-throughput assay for small molecules that modulate zebrafish embryonic heart rate. Nature Chemical Biology. 2005;**1**:263-264

[103] Chitramuthu BP. Modeling human disease and development in zebrafish. Human Genet Embryology. 2013;**3**:e108. DOI: 10.4172/2161-0436.1000e108

[104] Gama Sosa MA, De Gasperi R, Elder GA. Modeling human neurodegenerative diseases in transgenic systems. Human Genetics. 2012;**131**:535-563

[105] Berman J, Payne E, Hall C. The zebrafish as a tool to study hematopoiesis, human blood diseases, and immune function. Advances in Hematology. 2012;**2012**:2. Article ID 425345. https://doi.org/10.1155/2012/425345

[106] Brownlie A, Donovan A, Pratt SJ, Paw BH, Oates AC, et al. Positional cloning of the zebrafish sauternes gene: A model for congenital sideroblastic anaemia. Nature Genetics. 1998;**20**:244-250

[107] Sehnert AJ, Huq A, Weinstein BM, Walker C, Fishman M, et al. Cardiac troponin T is essential in sarcomere assembly and cardiac contractility. Nature Genetics. 2002;**31**:106-110

[108] Lin YY. Muscle diseases in the zebrafish. Neuromuscular Disorders. 2012;**22**:673-684

[109] Liu S, Leach SD. Zebrafish models for cancer. Annual Review of Pathology. 2011;**6**:71-93

[110] Patton EE, Widlund HR, Kutok JL, Kopani KR, Amatruda JF, et al. BRAF mutations are sufficient to promote nevi formation and cooperate with p53 in the genesis of melanoma. Current Biology. 2005;**15**:249-254

[111] Sarath Babu N, Murthy CLN, Kakara S, Sharma R, Swamy B, Cherukuvada V, et al. 1-Methyl-4-phenyl-1, 2,3, 6-tetrahydropyridine induced Parkinson's disease in zebrafish. Proteomics. 2016;**16**:1407-1420

[112] Chakravarty S, Reddy BR, Sudhakar SR, Saxena S, Das T, Meghah V, et al. Chronic unpredictable stress (CUS)-induced anxiety and related mood disorders in a zebrafish model: Altered brain proteome profile implicates mitochondrial dysfunction. PLoS One. 2013;**8**:e63302

[113] Dahm R, Geisler R. Learning from small fry: The zebrafish as a genetic model organism for aquaculture fish species. Marine Biotechnology. 2006;**8**(4):329-345

[114] Van der Sar AM, Appelmelk BJ, Vandenbroucke-Grauls CM, Bitter W. A star with stripes: Zebrafish as an infection model. Trends in Microbiology. 2004;**12**:451-457

Chapter 2

Immunotherapy for Treatment of Cancer

Aida Karachi

Abstract

Cancer is known to be second cause of death worldwide despite aggressive therapeutic measures such as surgical resection of tumors, radiation therapy, and chemotherapy. The failure of currently available therapeutics for cancers, has led to increasing interest in alternative approaches including immunotherapy. Immunotherapy for cancer treatment is enhancing immune responses to fight cancer cells. Monoclonal antibodies, immune checkpoint blockades, targeted therapy, adoptive cell therapy, CAR T cells, and cancer vaccines are the most current and efficient parts of immunotherapy armamentarium. Immunotherapy has tremendous success in the treatment of cancers and is considered as a standard care of treatment or recurrence preventive therapy for variety of cancers. In this chapter, we discuss different types of immunotherapy for cancer treatment in detail.

Keywords: immunotherapy, immune checkpoint blockades, cancer vaccines, adoptive cell therapy, CAR T cell, personalized immunotherapy

1. Introduction

Cancer is the second most common cause of death in the world that has threatened health for thousands of years. Several aggressive measures such as surgical resection of tumors, chemotherapy, and radiotherapy are used to cure cancers. Although these therapeutics can minimize and inhibit cancer cells proliferation and metastasis, they have not been able to effectively defeat cancers until now. The efficacy of conventional treatments for cancer management is limited by factors such as recurrence of tumors and severe toxicities induced by therapeutics. Immunotherapy has become a tempting approach a long time after William Coley described the first immune stimulation by live bacteria for the treatment of cancer in 1893 [1]. Immunotherapy harnesses patients' own immune system to kill cancer cells thereby reducing toxic effects of traditional chemotherapy and radiotherapy. Immune cells can identify cancer cells by recognizing tumor-associated antigens. The ability of cancer cells to escape from immune system has limited the efficacy of immunotherapy. Current novel approaches have been involved in immunotherapy to stop immune evasion of cancer cells.

Immunotherapy includes several therapies such as monoclonal antibodies, tumor cell vaccines, immune cell vaccines, and adoptive cell therapy. Monoclonal antibodies, which block cytotoxic T lymphocyte-associated protein-4 (CTLA-4), programmed cell death-1 (PD-1), dendritic cell vaccines, and chimeric antigen receptor (CAR) T cells have shown a tremendous success in clinical trials for several cancers. It is shown that immunotherapy has the potential to move to the front-line of therapeutic options in most cancers. Despite the benefits of immunotherapy, some treatments have severe side effects such as nausea, fever, and diarrhea [2]. The aim of this chapter is to study the concept of immunotherapy for cancer treatment and to provide a thorough review on immunotherapy's developments for both oncologists and cancer immunologists.

2. Monoclonal antibodies

One of the mechanisms of immune system to defeat pathogens or cancers is to identify foreign substances or malignancies and generate antibodies against them. These antibodies can recognize pathogens and cancer cells by the antigens expressed on their surface. Antibodies have the ability to attach to the specific antigens and destroy foreign particles or malignancies. In the laboratory, scientists can generate many copies of antibodies that are specific to certain antigens on cancer cells. These are known as monoclonal antibodies. In 1997, the first monoclonal antibody, rituximab, was approved for treatment of non-Hodgkin's lymphoma. Beneficial outcomes of rituximab treatment resulted in emergence and development of monoclonal antibodies as a therapeutic approach for various hematological and solid cancers [3]. The most important step in generating monoclonal antibodies for cancer treatment is identifying right antigens on cancer cells. High mutation capacity of cancer cells and existence of various antigens make this task challenging. So far, monoclonal antibodies therapy has been more beneficial against some cancers than others.

Monoclonal antibodies can defeat cancer in different ways. Some monoclonal antibodies can recognize antigens expressed by cancer cells and mark them as a target that should be destroyed by immune system. This monoclonal antibody treatment is also known as targeted therapy [4]. Some of monoclonal antibodies cause apoptosis in cancer cells by directly attaching to the cancer cells. Preventing cell proliferation, destroying cell membrane, delivering radiation or chemotherapy to cancer cells, and inhibiting blood vessel growth are other functions of monoclonal antibodies to stop cancer cells. Monoclonal antibodies can robust, mimic or maintain the immune system's response on cancer cells in different ways, and some particular monoclonal antibodies act by more than one function [3]. Monoclonal antibodies can be categorized to three groups such as naked monoclonal antibodies (**Table 1**), conjugated monoclonal antibodies (**Table 2**), and bispecific monoclonal antibodies. Naked monoclonal antibodies act by just a single function. This single function can either be directly affecting cancer cells or by improving immune system against cancer cells. Trastuzumab is an example of monoclonal antibodies with direct effect on cancer cells. Trastuzumab can identify and block HER2 antigen, which is highly expressed on breast and stomach cancer cells. HER2 antigen is responsible for growth and proliferation of cancer cells. By blocking HER2 antigens, cancer cells are not able to expand and proliferate and spread in the body [5]. Immune check point inhibitors are monoclonal antibodies which improve immune system function. This group of antibodies will be discussed in detail later on this chapter. Some monoclonal antibodies can trigger immune system by attaching to immune cells and activating immune cells to destroy cancer cells. Alemtuzumab, which is a monoclonal antibody to treat chronic lymphocytic leukemia, binds to CD25 marker on the surface of lymphocytes and attracts immune cells to destroy cancer cells [6]. Conjugated monoclonal antibodies, also known as tagged antibodies or loaded antibodies, are antibodies that are being used to deliver either chemotherapy drugs or radioactive particles to cancer cells. These monoclonal

Monoclonal antibody	Target	Type	Approval year	Cancer
Rituximab	CD20	Chimeric IgG1	1997	B cell non-Hodgkin lymphoma
Trastuzumab	EGF	Humanized IgG1	1998	Breast cancer
Gemtuzumab Ozogamicin	CD33		2000	Acute myeloid leukemia
Alemtuzumab	CD52	Humanized IgG1	2001	B cell chronic lymphocytic leukemia
Ibritumomab Tiuxetan	CD20		2002	B cell non-Hodgkin lymphoma
Cetuximab	VEGFR	Chimeric IgG1	2004	Merkel cell carcinoma
Bevacizumab	VEGF	Humanized IgG1	2004	Colon cancer
Panitumumab	EGFR	Human IgG2	2006	Colorectal Ca
Catumaxomab	CD3	Chimeric mouse-rat hybrid	2009	Malignant ascites
Ofatumumab	CD20	Human IgG1	2009	B cell chronic lymphocytic leukemia
Ipilimumab	CTLA-4	Human IgG1	2011	Melanoma
Brentuximab Vedotin	CD30		2011	Hodgkin lymphoma
Pertuzumab	HER2	Humanized IgG1	2012	Breast cancer
Ado-Trastuzumab Emtansine	HER2	Humanized IgG1	2013	Breast cancer
Obinutuzumab	CD20		2013	B cell chronic lymphocytic leukemia
Denosumab		Human IgG2	2013	Osteoclastoma
Ramucirumab	VEGFR2	Human IgG1	2014	Gastric Ca
Pembrolizumab	PD-1	Humanized IgG1	2014	Melanoma
Nivolumab	PD-1	Human IgG1	2014	Melanoma
Dinutuximab	GD2	Chimeric IgG1	2015	Neuroblastoma
Daratumumab	CD38	Human IgG1	2015	Multiple myeloma
Necitumumab	EGFR	Human IgG1	2015	Lung cancer
Elotuzumab	SLAMF7	Humanized IgG1	2015	Multiple myeloma
Atezolizumab	PD-L1	Humanized IgG1	2016	Urothelial cancer
Avelumab (14)	PD-L1	human IgG1 monoclonal antibody	2017	Metastatic merkel cell carcinoma
Durvalumab	PD-L1	human IgG1 kappa monoclonal antibody	2018	Urothelial carcinoma/ non-small cell lung cancer

Table 1.
Unconjugated monoclonal antibodies currently approved by the Food and Drug Administration (FDA) for cancer therapy.

antibodies reduce the toxic effects of systemic chemotherapy and radiotherapy by directly homing the toxic drugs to tumor microenvironment [7, 8]. Ibritumomab tiuxetan is a radio-immunotherapeutic drug which directly delivers radio isotopes to cancerous B cells in non-Hodgkin lymphoma. Ibritumomab tiuxetan is a radio-labeled monoclonal antibody against CD20 antigen, which is expressed on B cell surface. By attaching Ibritumomab tiuxetan to CD20 on the B cells and killing cancer cells, the drug is able to eliminate lymphoma [7]. Chemolabeled antibodies are monoclonal antibodies that are attached to chemotherapy drugs. Brentuximab

Monoclonal antibody	Target	Type	Approval year	Cancers
Ibritumomab tiuxetan	CD20 Radionucleotide (Yttrium^{90} or Indium^{111})	Murine IgG1	2002	B cell non-Hodgkin's lymphoma/ lymphoproliferative disorder
Ositumomab	CD20 Radionucleotide (Iodine^{131})	Murine IgG2a	2003	Non-Hodgkin lymphoma
Brentuximab vedotin	CD30	Chimeric IgG1 Drug (auristatin E)	2011	Hodgkin lymphoma and systemic anaplastic large cell lymphoma
Trastuzumab emtansine	Trastuzumab DM1	Humanized IgG1 Drug (mertansine)	2013	Breast cancer
Tositumomab; Iodine I 131 Tositumomab	CD19+ CD3	Murine IgG2a	2014	Acute lymphoblastic leukemia
Arcitumomab	Diagnostic	Murine IgG1		Colorectal cancer
Capromab pendetide	Diagnostic	Murine IgG1		Prostate cancer

Table 2.
Conjugated monoclonal antibodies currently approved by the Food and Drug Administration (FDA) for cancer therapy.

vedotin is a chemolabeled monoclonal antibody specific for CD30 antigen on lymphocytes that delivers monomethyl auristatin E chemotherapy to cancer cells for treatment of Hodgkin lymphoma and anaplastic large cell lymphoma [9]. Ado-trastuzumab emtansine is another chemolabeled antibody attached to Mertansine (DM1) chemotherapy with ability to target HER2 molecules on breast cancer cells [10]. Immunotoxin monoclonal antibodies are a new class of monoclonal antibodies that are attached to highly toxic protein molecules of a plant or bacteria. Immunotoxins can specifically bind to their target and deliver potent toxins to cancer cells [11]. The most recent group of antibodies is bispecific monoclonal antibodies that consist of two separate antibodies targeting different specific antigens. Blinatumomab is a bispecific monoclonal antibody with the ability to bind to CD19 on lymphoma and leukemia cells and CD3 on T cells. This antibody is usually used for treatment of acute lymphocytic leukemia. By binding to two antigens on separate cells, Blinatumomab is able to bring immune cells and cancer cells together and ease the pathway for immune cells to find, attack, and kill cancer cells [12].

Based on the genetically engineering techniques, four groups of monoclonal antibodies have been developed. Murine monoclonal antibodies, which were derived from mice, were the first generation of antibodies. They were quickly eliminated from clinical studies as they were not able to interact with human immune system. Chimeric monoclonal antibodies are another category of monoclonal antibodies, consist of constant regions mostly derived from human source and variable regions entirely derived from murine source [13]. There is a subtype of chimeric non-humanized monoclonal antibodies also known as rat-mouse hybrid monoclonal antibodies with murine Fc portion that have specificities for binding to three different tumor cells, T cells and also accessory cells [14]. On the other hand, chimeric humanized monoclonal antibodies, that comprise human Fc portion, are developed with more efficient interaction with human immune system and less immunogenicity [15]. Less immunogenic and more efficient monoclonal antibodies have been developed as humanized monoclonal antibodies, which predominantly originated from human source excluding Fab portion which is derived from murine source. Human monoclonal antibodies that are fully human and are derived from transgenic mice known to be the most efficient and the least immunogenic [16].

Although monoclonal antibodies are being used for treatment of cancer, they may increase the risk of immune reactions or adverse effects. The immune reactions including acute anaphylactic reaction, serum sickness, or cytokine release syndrome (CRS) generally occur after first infusion of monoclonal antibodies. Adverse effects of monoclonal antibodies are the result of immunodeficiency mediated by blockade of specific targets. Infections such as reactivation of tuberculosis or progressive multifocal leukoencephalopathy, autoimmune diseases such as lupus and thyroid disease, cancer, dermatitis, and organ-specific adverse effects are other risks of monoclonal antibodies administration [13]. The other problem of monoclonal antibodies are constant mutation of cancer cells which results in formation of different or neoantigens that already available antibodies cannot function against them. Generation of different or neoantigens lead to absence of responsiveness to monoclonal antibodies. Developed genome sequencing techniques is promising for identifying neoantigens and producing monoclonal antibodies against this targets [3]. Monoclonal antibodies have been proven to remarkably shrink solid tumors, suppress malignancies, diminish metastasis, and increase overall survival in patients [17, 18]. Monoclonal antibodies are promising for treatment of cancers in both monotherapy and in combinatorial therapeutic approaches.

3. Immune checkpoint blockades

It was believed that cancer cells were completely resistant to immune system till 1800s when researchers reported regression or total elimination of some solid tumors in patients who had streptococcal skin infections or were infused with bacterial extracts [1, 19]. These studies were not continued until Sharma and Allison noticed that blocking of cytotoxic T lymphocyte-associated protein 4 (CTLA-4) enhances tumor killing capacity of T cells [20]. This hypothesis pops up that some bacterial or organisms' extracts have the ability to block molecules on immune cells, known as checkpoints, which promote immune cells' functionality against cancer cells. These observations led to more in-depth studies to identify immune checkpoints which their blockade can trigger robust anticancer immune responses.

One type of monoclonal antibodies that bind to immune check points is referred as immune checkpoint blockades. Checkpoints or coinhibitory receptors are molecules on immune cells that bind to their ligands expressed on normal cells. Under normal circumstances, immune checkpoints recognize healthy cells as non-pathogenic by binding to the ligands on normal cells and prevent activity of the immune system against its own tissue. Some cancer cells express check points ligands which help them to escape from recognition and elimination by immune system. By blocking immune checkpoints, immune cells gain a robust response against cancer cells. Immune check point blockades have been proven to be effective in many cancers and are promising because they are targeting immune cells by removing inhibitory pathways [21].

CTLA-4 is a coinhibitory receptor on T cells that prevent T cells activation. During T cells activation, antigen-presenting cells (APCs) present processed antigens on their major histocompatibility complex (MHC) molecules to T cell receptors. After the initial phase of activation, B7-1 or B7-2 molecules of APCs attach to CD28 on T cells. TCR signal and costimulatory B7-CD28 induce complete T cell activation that result in cytokine release from activated T cells [22]. Besides, inhibitory signals induce by CTLA-4 act in an opposite way [23]. CTLA-4 molecule expressed on T cells has a higher affinity to bind to B7 compare to CD28. In a competition between CD28 and CTLA-4, CTLA-4 predominantly binds to B7 and generates an inhibitory signal during T cells activation. Inhibitory signals of CTLA-4 halt T cells activation and induce immune tolerance. Blocking of CTLA-4 by Ipilimumab (CTLA-4 blockade) was first approved by FDA due to success of CTLA-4 blockade in treatment of melanoma patients [24]. Ipilimumab boosts immune responses to cancer cells mediated by T cells activation. Most of patients experience Ipilimumab-related side effects like diarrhea, vomiting, skin rashes, nausea, and even life-threatening effects. All patients receiving this drug are always monitored closely and side effects are managed by corticosteroids [25].

In cancer, T cells are constantly exposed to antigen stimulation which result in gradual deterioration of their function by losing cytokine production ability and persistent increase in expression of inhibitory receptors. Defects in T cell activation, cytokine production, and proliferation is defined as exhaustion. Inhibitory receptors are highly expressed on exhausted T cells. Cancer cells have a high expression of inhibitory ligands that increase the chance of exhaustion in T cells. Programmed cell death-1 (PD-1) is an inhibitory molecule known as the receptor for cell death and have regulatory inhibitory role in activation of T cells. Physiologically, PD-1/PD-1 ligand (PD-L1) signaling pathway is a way to control excessive inflammation to protect normal tissues by induction of immune tolerance [26]. Interaction of PD-1 and PD-L1, which is highly expressed on tumor cells, causes exhaustion and dysfunctionality in T cells that avoid immune response against cancer cells. PD-1 or PD-L1 inhibitors pharmacologically prevent interaction of these molecules and efficiently maintain T cells function and facilitate them to kill tumor cells. Both PD-1 and PD-L1 immune checkpoint blockades have been proven to be effective for many malignancies but still it is not obvious that whether blocking of PD-1 on T cells or PD-L1 on tumors is more effective for cancer treatment. Patients' characteristics such as type of tumor, mutation burden of tumor, and metastases of tumor affect efficacy of PD-1/PD-L1 inhibitors [27]. PD-L1 is not constantly expressed on different tumors and even in different stages of tumor growth. Therefore, efficacy of PD-L1 blockade depends on the type of tumor, stage of tumor, location of the tumor, and many other factors [28, 29]. Atezolizumab, the first FDA-approved PD-L1 blockade, has been used as the first-line treatment of metastatic non-small lung carcinoma and cisplatin-resistant metastatic urothelial carcinoma. Avelumab, is another FDA-approved PD-L1 blockade for metastatic merkel cell carcinoma that lack efficient response to chemotherapy [30]. Nivolumab and Pembrolizumab are PD-1 blockers and are successfully used in Phase I clinical trial on patients with non-small-cell lung cancer and renal cell carcinoma. Nivolumab was approved by FDA for treatment of advanced melanoma patients after significant improved response in phase III trial. Also, Pembrolizumab is the first-line immune checkpoint blockade for the treatment of metastatic melanoma and metastatic non-small cell lung cancer [31]. These drugs have significantly increased survival of patients with minimal side effects in other solid tissue tumors. To improve benefits from immune checkpoint blockades, combinatorial strategies are under study. Combination regimens include administration of two immune checkpoint blockades together or a monoclonal antibody with chemotherapy or radiotherapy [32]. Combinatorial strategies enhance anticancer responses because each treatment works through targeting different pathways. Combination therapy of Ipilimumab/Nivolumab is approved by FDA for treatment of melanoma [33]. Pembrolizumab plus chemotherapy (pemetrexed/carboplatin) is approved for treatment of non-small cell lung carcinoma [34]. Several combination therapies including either two different checkpoint blockades or with chemo/radiotherapy are under investigation [32].

Immune checkpoint blockades have changed the treatment strategies for cancer with dramatic improves in many cancers. PD-1, PD-L1, and CTLA-4 inhibitors are able to change immune responses and it may cause adverse immune reactions. These immune reactions are usually better tolerated than chemotherapy drugs but still recognition and proactive treatments should be included in the treatment strategy for patients receiving immune checkpoint blockades [35].

4. Cancer vaccines

Cancer vaccines are a new generation of vaccines different to traditional prophylactic vaccines which were administered to healthy people. Cancer vaccines are administered to either prevent cancer in high-risk individuals or to treat cancer in patients with malignancies. Therapeutic cancer vaccines are able to enhance immune system to attack cancer cells. Two prophylactic vaccines were approved for cancers that are caused by virus infections. One of the prophylactic vaccines is for hepatitis B virus (HBV) infection that can cause liver cancers such as cirrhosis and hepatocellular carcinoma in those who suffer from chronic infections. Another prophylactic vaccine is against human papilloma virus (HPV) that mediates cervical, anal, vaginal, vulvar, and throat cancers as well as genital warts. Until now, preventive vaccines were only available for the cancers that are caused by infections. Therapeutic vaccines are meant to enhance immune system in order to interfere with cancer cells, stop their growth and proliferation, and kill cancer cells. Therapeutic cancers are divided to several categories of cell vaccines, peptide vaccines, and genetic vaccines.

Tumor cell vaccines are a type of cell vaccines including autologous tumor cell vaccines and allogenic tumor cell vaccines. Autologous tumor cell vaccines are isolated from patient-derived tumor cells and prepared in vitro for administration to the patient from whom the tumor cells were isolated. Preparation of tumor cells for vaccination includes irradiation of tumor cells or combining tumor cells with an immune stimulatory adjuvant such as recombinant granulocyte monocyte-colony stimulating factor (GM-CSF) [36]. Autologous cell vaccines are able to present a wide range of tumor-associated antigens to cytotoxic T cells, resulting in a robust antitumor activity. Modification of autologous tumor cells to induce higher levels of immune stimulation has been studied by many researchers. Autologous tumor cell vaccines in animal tumor models of lymphoma and melanoma were more potent when tumor cell vaccines were infected with Newcastle disease virus [37]. In another study, tumor cell vaccines were genetically modified to express higher levels of IL-2 which induced activation of T cells and natural killer (NK) cells [38]. Autologous tumor cell vaccines transduced with GM-CSF, named GVAX, are able to get involved with dendritic cells (DCs), and induce maturation of DCs. GVAX-mediated matured DCs activate cytotoxic T cells and improve T cells response to cancer [39]. Autologous tumor cell vaccines have been extensively investigated in clinical and preclinical studies on several cancers and approximately 20% of patients survived for a long time [40]. The advantage of autologous tumor cell vaccines is that the vaccines can target the patient's own tumor-associated antigens and excludes the step to select specific antigens. One major problem in preparing autologous tumor cell vaccines is the time-consuming process of harvesting sufficient amount of tumor cells, which is a restriction for certain tumors. Appose to autologous tumor cell vaccines, allogeneic tumor cell vaccines are easy and less expensive to produce in large scales. Allogeneic whole tumor cell vaccines consist of at least two human tumor cell lines and have unlimited tumor-specific antigens. Canavaxin is an allogeneic tumor cell vaccine consisting of three irradiated allogeneic melanoma cell lines combined with adjuvant Bacillus Calmette-Guérin (BCG). Despite Canavaxin increased overall survival of melanoma patients in phase II of trials, clinical trials were terminated because of failure of the vaccine in stages III and IV [41]. Allogeneic GVAX vaccine has been studied for treatment of prostate cancer [42], breast cancer [43], and pancreatic cancer [44]. Combination of GVAX vaccine with CTLA-4 antibody (Ipilimumab) was approved by FDA for treatment of metastatic melanoma [45]. Belagenpumatucel-L is another allogeneic tumor cell vaccine formed from four non-small cell lung carcinoma (NSCLC) cell lines transfected with plasmid containing a transforming growth factor (TGF)-beta2 antisense transgene. This genetically modified vaccine secretes TGF-beta and is used for treatment of NSCLC [46].

5. Dendritic cell vaccines

Dendritic cell (DC) vaccines emerged as a potent cancer vaccine. DCs are professional antigen-presenting cells (APCs) that act as a bridge between innate and adoptive immune system [47]. DCs uptake pathogens, process them, and present pathogen antigens on their MHC molecules. Processed antigens on DCs are directly recognized by T cells which induce antigen-specific immune responses. Different subtypes of DCs exist in human body based on CD8, CD103, or CD11b expressions. DCs are in both non-lymphoid organs and lymphoid organs such as lymph nodes, spleens, and bone marrow. Classical DCs (cDCs) are divided to CD8+, CD103+, and CD11b+ DCs. Non-classic DCs include monocyte-derived DCs, plasmacytoid DCs, and Langerhans cells. These categories are based on expression of molecules and the location of DCs in body [48]. Studies showed that different subsets of DCs can prime and expand various T cells. For example, CD8+ CD205+ DCs present antigens on both MHC-I and MHC-II and are able to prime CD4+ T cell and CD8+ T cells but CD8-33D1+ DCs present antigens just on MHC-II and prime CD4+ T cells [49]. DCs act as a double-edged sword that can induce both immune tolerance and immune activation depending on which receptors on DCs are engaged [50]. Maturation and migration of DCs play a critical role in characteristics of DCs [51]. Matured DCs migrate to lymphoid organs and prime T cells to enhance antitumor responses. Loading of MHC molecules with cancer antigens, up regulation of costimulatory molecules such as CD40, CD80, and CD86 on DCs, and cytokine production of DCs are critically required for activation of T cells DCs [52, 53]. DC vaccines include ex vivo generation of DCs from CD34+ hematopoietic progenitor cells or peripheral blood-derived monocytes (PBMC) [53]. Ex vivo-generated DCs are loaded with appropriate source of tumor antigens and are subsequently activated with adjuvants and are administered back to patients to kill tumors. Tumor antigens derived from total tumor [54], DNA/RNA virus [55], tumor proteins, or peptides [56, 57] are utilized for DC vaccines. Moreover, some DC vaccines are composed of fusion of tumor cells and ex vivo-generated DCs [58]. Autologous DC vaccine pulsed with HLA-A0201 peptide (prostate-specific antigen) was among the first dendritic cell vaccines used in clinical trials with promising results [56]. DC vaccines have been studies in many clinical trials on various cancers. FDA-approved Sipuleucel-T DC vaccine for the first time for the treatment of metastatic castrate-resistant prostate cancer [59]. Sipuleucel-T composed of PBMC-derived DCs loaded with PA2024 (prostatic acid phosphate) fused to GM-CSF, which significantly increased patients survival. Although DC vaccines were successful in prostate cancer treatment, their efficacy in other cancers was modest. Researchers conduct studies to enhance DC vaccines potency by modulating stimulatory and inhibitory molecules on DCs. Modulation of costimulatory molecules such as CD40L, CD70, GITRL, CD137L, and OX40L [60–63] or inflammatory markers of IL-12p70, IL-18, IL-12, CXCL10, and CCR7 on DCs improve DCs maturation and T cell priming characteristics [64–68]. The other way to enhance anticancer T cell response by DCs is to suppress inhibitory molecules on DCs. Genetically silencing of ubiquitin-editing enzyme A20 [69], suppressor of cytokine signaling 1 (SOCS1) [70], and scavenger receptor SRA/CD204 [71] improve DCs function and subsequently enhance T cell response to cancer cells.

Two of the most important limitations of cancer cell vaccines and DC vaccines are limited source of specimen and complicated procedure to generate these vaccines. New vaccines generated by tumor-associated antigen peptides combined with an adjuvant seemed to solve the restrictions of cancer cell and DC vaccines. The first encoded human tumor-associated antigen peptide was named MAGE-1 [72]. Different types of tumor-associated antigen peptides are studied. Cancer testis antigens are a group of genes available in both healthy and cancerous tissues. These genes such as MAGE, BAGE, NY-ESO-1, and SSX-2 are scant in normal tissues but are highly expressed in tumors [73–75]. Tissue differentiation antigens are available and active in both healthy tissues and tumors-like PSA and PAP in prostate cancer [76, 77], gp100, Melan-A/Mart-1, and tyrosinase in melanoma [78–80], and mammaglobin-A in breast carcinomas [81]. Tumor-specific antigens or -mutated oncogenes are a group of antigens expressed on both normal tissues and tumors with a unique up regulation in tumors such as CEA [82], MUC-1 [83], HER2/Neu [84], and certain antiapoptotic proteins (i.e. livin and survivin) [85, 86]. Clinical trials mostly focused on effects of peptide vaccines that target cancer testis antigens, and differentiation-associated antigens. To produce an effective peptide vaccine, addition of immune stimulatory adjuvant is required for an efficient immune response as tumor-associated antigens are not immunogenic. Some adjuvants used for peptide vaccine generation are aluminum salt, pathogen-associated molecular patterns (PAMPs), TLR agonists [87], BCG [88], and monophosphoryl lipid A (MPL) [89]. Cervarix is the first peptide vaccine for human papillomavirus composed of MPL and aluminum salt [90]. The advantage of peptide vaccines to DC vaccines and cancer cell vaccines is that peptide vaccines are more cost effective, but they may also appear to be less potent because they only target one or few epitopes of tumor-associated antigens. Formulation of peptide vaccines, route of delivery, and selection of immunogenic adjuvants can influence efficacy of peptide vaccines [91].

6. Genetic vaccines

Genetic vaccines are another approach for carrying tumor-associated antigens to patients by utilizing plasmid DNA vectors. Genetic vaccines transfect DCs and directly present tumor-associated antigens to cytotoxic T cells or they can transfect somatic cells and indirectly cross prime T cells. Each genetic vaccine can deliver many tumor-associated antigens to patients and induce a robust anticancer immunity [92]. DNA vaccines are composed of bacterial plasmids that carry genes of interest under the control of mammalian promoter. DNA vaccines are able to initiate innate immunity and based on the site of delivery, they can trigger cellular and humoral immunity [93]. Usually the transgene is cytomegalovirus (CMV) immediate early promoter and its intron A sequence [94]. Optimizing codon usage can increase the transduction of antigens. In the intra muscular administration of DNA vaccines, DNA plasmids transfect both myocytes and DCs. The plasmids act as an immunogenic and activate T cells via toll-like receptors [95]. DNA sensors in cytosol of cells such as DAI, H2B, IFI16, DDX41, LRRFIP1, and cGAS are able to detect presence of DNA vaccines. DNA sensors send signal to STING-TBK1 signaling cascade and activate interferon regulatory factor 3 which results in expression of type I interferons. TLR9 recognizes unmethylated CpG DNA and activates interferon regulatory factor 7 that induce expression of interferons. DCs phagocyte antigen-expressing cell (myocytes) and cross present antigens on MHC-I to CD8 T cells. Moreover, interferons promote this pathway. If DNA vaccines directly transfect DCs, DCs are able to uptake, process, and present antigens on MHC-I to CD8 T cells [96]. Transfection of the vector with multiple gene sequences increases the immunization and induces humoral [97] and CD8 T cell response [98]. Combination of DC vaccines with other immune stimulatory agents such as TLR agonists [99], or monoclonal antibodies [100] increase anticancer immunity. RNA vaccines are safe vaccines compared to DNA vaccines as they degrade and clear quickly in body. Total tumor RNAs are isolated from tumor tissues and they can induce a potent immune response. RNA vaccines are composed of various tumor antigens which reduce the possibility of immune escape by tumor cells. The first use of RNA vaccines was to immunize patients with mRNAs that encode tumor-associated antigens. Furthermore, RNA vaccines can be produced for personalized cancer treatment. Patients' neoantigens can be identified by tumor exome analyzing and personalized RNA vaccine can be specifically generated. In addition to direct use of mRNAs for vaccine generation, RNAs are utilized in cell therapies. Transfecting patient-derived cells with RNAs and giving manipulated cells back to patients are another form of utilizing mRNAs. For example, transfection of patient-derived DCs with mRNA of tumor-associated antigens can induce an antigen-specific T cell response in cancer patients. Transfection of patient-derived T cells with mRNA of chimeric antigen receptors, triggers T cells to identify specific antigens on cancer cells which quickly deteriorate cancer [101]. Liposomes and protaminase are adjuvants of RNA vaccines and help to stabilize RNAs [102].

7. Adoptive cell therapy

Adoptive T cell therapy (ACT) is a treatment that enhances T cells' ability to kill cancer cells by transferring immune system-derived cells to patients. The cells used for ACT can originate from the same patient or another individual. In 1988, the first ACT reduced metastatic melanoma tumors with transferring of autologous CD4+ and CD8+ tumor infiltrating lymphocytes (TILs) to the patients [103, 104]. Both peripheral blood T cells and TILs extracted from tumors are utilized to generate specific T cells for ACT. These T cells can be modified and then transferred to patients or directly administered in their natural state. TILs by their own nature have an antitumor activity as they are specific for tumor cells. TILs can recognize tumor antigens such as cancer germline antigens, neoantigens, and viral proteins and kill cancer cells [104]. After tumors are resected, the tumor tissues digest into fragments and each fragment is cultured in the presence of IL-2. The T cells are expanded and each clone is monitored for its reactivity against tumor cells. Proliferating lymphocytes kill tumor cells and produce a pure population of T cells. Cancer reactive T cells are infused back to patients. Moreover, T cells that express a TCR specific for tumor antigens can be selected in vitro from peripheral blood and expanded. Antigen-specific T cells are selected by coculturing of T cells with APCs loaded with tumor particles such as RNAs. By expansion of antigen-specific T cells, a specific antitumor T cell clone can be generated [105]. T cells with TCR targeting tumorigenic mutations such as Ras mutations have shown promise in cancer treatment. Ras is commonly mutated at the onset of tumorigenesis in the dominant population of tumor cells. Targeting Ras mutations and killing tumor cells with Ras-specific ACT may have profound effects on cancers with Ras mutations [106]. TCRs targeting KRAS G12D, a common proto-oncogene encoding GTPase, have anti-tumorigenic effects on patients with colorectal cancer [107]. Also, genetically modified antitumor T cell clones can be produced by infecting T cells with viruses that carry genetically engineered TCRs [108]. TCR-transduced T cells are generated by cloning specific TCRs into a retrovirus. Patients derived PBMCs are activated with CD3 and IL-2 and are transduced with the retrovirus encoding the antigen-specific TCR. The T cells are expanded and injected back to the individuals. Peripheral blood T cells transfected with retrovirus encoding MART-1 TCR regress tumors in melanoma [103]. Genetically engineering techniques can modify TCRs to target-specific antigens. For example, T cells with modified TCRs that target NY-ESO-1, a cancer germline antigen, were successfully used as ACT for treatment of patients with synovial cell sarcoma and melanoma [109]. One major limitation of ACTs is that they induce short-lasting responses in immune system. Administration of T cells after chemotherapy increases cancer regression due to repopulation of host T cells with antigen-specific T cells. Lymphodepletion induced by chemotherapy helps T cells from ACT to proliferate during hemostatic proliferative phase and persist for months after infusion [109]. It was also shown that high doses of IL-2 therapy contribute to expansion of the transferred cells [110, 111]. The first signal in T cell activation begins with binding of TCR to MHC molecules on APCs. Furthermore, MHC expression downregulates on APCs in cancers so that they can escape immunity [112]. In 1989, first chimeric antigen receptors (CARs) were developed to avoid interaction of T cells with MHC molecules. CAR T cells are designed to identify cancer cells and attack them without mediation of APCs. As a result, CARs act independent of any stimulatory and TCR signaling. CAR composed of a ligand-binding domain and a signaling domain. Ligand-binding domain is the extracellular part of CAR that includes B cell receptor derived single chain variable fragment. The signaling domain is made of costimulatory molecules and CD3f and 1 [112]. CD19 CAR T cells were used in clinical trial for patients with refractory B cell lymphoma and hematological malignancies. No acute graft versus host disease (GVHD) has been reported in patients except for one mild chronic ocular GVHD that was observed 2 years after CAR T cells infusion [113]. In 2017, FDA-approved Tisagenlecleucel, CD19 CAR T cell, for the treatment of acute lymphoblastic leukemia (ALL). Excellent results with these trials, increased interests in CAR T cell immunotherapy approach [114, 115]. Cytokine release syndrome (CRS) is one of the side effects of CAR T Cells. CRS is a storm of inflammatory cytokines including IL-6, IL-10, and IFN-γ that happens after the infusion of CAR T cells [2]. Patients may show symptoms such as hypotension, pulmonary edema, multi-organ failure, and even CRS-related death. Treatment of CRS includes administration of corticosteroids and IL-6 blockade. Using corticosteroids for treatment of CRS symptoms is controversial as corticosteroids dramatically decrease inflammatory cytokines and mitigate CAR T cells efficacy [116]. Another problem with CAR T cells is that they cannot penetrate into solid tumors. Studies are underway to alleviate limitations of CAR T cells and improve their efficacy for treatment of solid tumors [117].

8. Developing personalized immunotherapy

Many cancer patients do not benefit from immunotherapies they are receiving. Recently, many studies are focusing on identifying predictive and prognostic biomarkers in cancers as a beneficial guide for treatment decisions. This will stop administration of drugs for those patients who does not benefit from them and improve treatment in patients that are most likely respond to specific immunotherapies. Selecting the appropriate immunotherapy for each cancer patient is still a challenge. Scientists and oncologists are developing methods in genomic testing to discover cell signaling and biomarkers involved in responding to immunotherapy. It has been shown that cancers identified by specific quantity or pattern of mutations in the tumor microenvironment or surrounding area are more responsive to immune checkpoint blockades. Of note, scientists are trying to exploit other drugs to alter the tumor microenvironment of less immune responsive tumors, known as cold tumors, and turn them to check point blockades susceptible tumors that are defined as hot tumors [32]. Altering tumor microenvironment and surrounding tissues can increase the number of patients who can benefit from immune checkpoint blockades. Immunopharmacogenomics approach is providing a significant hope for personalized immunotherapy [118].

9. Conclusion

In summary, immunotherapy shows a tremendous potential in treatment of cancer. Different immunotherapies have been approved by FDA for prevention and treatment of cancers. Despite the breakthroughs achieved by immunotherapy, many cancers still do not respond to immunotherapy. Monotherapy of immune checkpoint blockades or other immunotherapies failed in treatment of some cancers. Finding the efficient treatment by combinatorial immunotherapies or combination of immunotherapy and traditional chemotherapy and radiotherapy are under investigation. Development of DCs and cancer vaccines, immune checkpoint blockades, CAR T cells, and ACT requires an in-depth understanding of tumor microenvironment and identifying tumor-specific antigens. More studies to develop immunotherapy can provide improved efficacy in cancer treatments.

Author details

Aida Karachi
UF Brain Tumor Immunotherapy Program, Lillian S. Wells Department of Neurosurgery, Preston A. Wells Jr. Center for Brain Tumor Therapy, University of Florida, Gainesville, FL, USA

*Address all correspondence to: aidakarachi@yahoo.com

References

[1] Coley WB. II. Contribution to the knowledge of sarcoma. Annals of Surgery. 1891;**14**(3):199-220

[2] Maude SL, Barrett D, Teachey DT, Grupp SA. Managing cytokine release syndrome associated with novel T cell-engaging therapies. Cancer Journal. 2014;**20**(2):119-122

[3] Coulson A, Levy A, Gossell-Williams M. Monoclonal antibodies in cancer therapy: Mechanisms, successes and limitations. The West Indian Medical Journal. 2014;**63**(6):650-654

[4] Vanneman M, Dranoff G. Combining immunotherapy and targeted therapies in cancer treatment. Nature Reviews. Cancer. 2012;**12**(4):237-251

[5] Pinto AC, Ades F, de Azambuja E, Piccart-Gebhart M. Trastuzumab for patients with HER2 positive breast cancer: Delivery, duration and combination therapies. Breast. 2013;**22**(Suppl 2):S152-S155

[6] Fiegl M, Stauder R, Steurer M, et al. Alemtuzumab in chronic lymphocytic leukemia: Final results of a large observational multicenter study in mostly pretreated patients. Annals of Hematology. 2014;**93**(2):267-277

[7] Steiner M, Neri D. Antibody-radionuclide conjugates for cancer therapy: Historical considerations and new trends. Clinical Cancer Research. 2011;**17**(20):6406-6416

[8] Flygare JA, Pillow TH, Aristoff P. Antibody-drug conjugates for the treatment of cancer. Chemical Biology & Drug Design. 2013;**81**(1):113-121

[9] Fanale MA, Horwitz SM, Forero-Torres A, et al. Brentuximab vedotin in the front-line treatment of patients with CD30+ peripheral T-cell lymphomas: Results of a phase I study. Journal of Clinical Oncology. 2014;**32**(28):3137-3143

[10] Amiri-Kordestani L, Blumenthal GM, Xu QC, et al. FDA approval: Ado-trastuzumab emtansine for the treatment of patients with HER2-positive metastatic breast cancer. Clinical Cancer Research. 2014;**20**(17):4436-4441

[11] Ehrlich D, Wang B, Lu W, Dowling P, Yuan R. Intratumoral anti-HuD immunotoxin therapy for small cell lung cancer and neuroblastoma. Journal of Hematology & Oncology. 2014;**7**:91

[12] Kaplan JB, Grischenko M, Giles FJ. Blinatumomab for the treatment of acute lymphoblastic leukemia. Investigational New Drugs. 2015;**33**(6):1271-1279

[13] Hansel TT, Kropshofer H, Singer T, Mitchell JA, George AJ. The safety and side effects of monoclonal antibodies. Nature Reviews. Drug Discovery. 2010;**9**(4):325-338

[14] Seimetz D. Novel monoclonal antibodies for cancer treatment: The trifunctional antibody catumaxomab (removab). Journal of Cancer. 2011;**2**:309-316

[15] Reichert JM, Rosensweig CJ, Faden LB, Dewitz MC. Monoclonal antibody successes in the clinic. Nature Biotechnology. 2005;**23**(9):1073-1078

[16] Lonberg N. Human monoclonal antibodies from transgenic mice. Handbook of Experimental Pharmacology. 2008;**181**:69-97

[17] Topalian SL, Sznol M, McDermott DF, et al. Survival, durable tumor remission, and long-term safety in patients with advanced melanoma receiving nivolumab. Journal of Clinical Oncology. 2014;**32**(10):1020-1030

[18] Naidoo J, Page DB, Li BT, et al. Toxicities of the anti-PD-1 and anti-PD-L1 immune checkpoint antibodies. Annals of Oncology. 2016;**27**(7):1362

[19] Littman DR. Releasing the brakes on cancer immunotherapy. Cell. 2015;**162**(6):1186-1190

[20] Sharma P, Allison JP. Immune checkpoint targeting in cancer therapy: Toward combination strategies with curative potential. Cell. 2015;**161**(2):205-214

[21] Tsai HF, Hsu PN. Cancer immunotherapy by targeting immune checkpoints: Mechanism of T cell dysfunction in cancer immunity and new therapeutic targets. Journal of Biomedical Science. 2017;**24**(1):35

[22] Fife BT, Bluestone JA. Control of peripheral T-cell tolerance and autoimmunity via the CTLA-4 and PD-1 pathways. Immunological Reviews. 2008;**224**:166-182

[23] Collins AV, Brodie DW, Gilbert RJ, et al. The interaction properties of costimulatory molecules revisited. Immunity. 2002;**17**(2):201-210

[24] Hodi FS, O'Day SJ, McDermott DF, et al. Improved survival with ipilimumab in patients with metastatic melanoma. The New England Journal of Medicine. 2010;**363**(8):711-723

[25] Camacho LH. CTLA-4 blockade with ipilimumab: Biology, safety, efficacy, and future considerations. Cancer Medicine. 2015;**4**(5): 661-672

[26] McDermott J, Jimeno A. Pembrolizumab: PD-1 inhibition as a therapeutic strategy in cancer. Drugs Today (Barc). 2015;**51**(1):7-20

[27] Ohaegbulam KC, Assal A, Lazar-Molnar E, Yao Y, Zang X. Human cancer immunotherapy with antibodies to the PD-1 and PD-L1 pathway. Trends in Molecular Medicine. 2015;**21**(1):24-33

[28] Mu L, Long Y, Yang C, et al. The IDH1 mutation-induced oncometabolite, 2-hydroxyglutarate, may affect DNA methylation and expression of PD-L1 in gliomas. Frontiers in Molecular Neuroscience. 2018;**11**:82

[29] Karachi A, Azari H, Flores C, Yang C, Dastmalchi F, Mitchell D, et al. TMZ results in priming of host immunity and changes in GBM tumor PDL-1 expression in a dose dependent fashion that can be leveraged for combination with immune checkpoint blockade: December 2016. Neuro-Oncology;**18**(Suppl 6):vi202

[30] Gaiser MR, Bongiorno M, Brownell I. PD-L1 inhibition with avelumab for metastatic Merkel cell carcinoma. Expert Review of Clinical Pharmacology. 2018;**11**(4):345-359

[31] Postow MA, Callahan MK, Wolchok JD. Immune checkpoint blockade in cancer therapy. Journal of Clinical Oncology. 2015;**33**(17):1974-1982

[32] Karachi A, Dastmalchi F, Mitchell D, Rahman M. Temozolomide for immunomodulation in the treatment of glioblastoma. Neuro-Oncology. 2018; noy072. https://doi.org/10.1093/neuonc/noy072

[33] Postow MA, Chesney J, Pavlick AC, et al. Nivolumab and ipilimumab versus ipilimumab in untreated melanoma. The New England Journal of Medicine. 2015;**372**(21):2006-2017

[34] Langer CJ, Gadgeel SM, Borghaei H, et al. Carboplatin and pemetrexed with or without pembrolizumab for advanced, non-squamous non-small-cell lung cancer: a randomised, phase 2 cohort of the open-label KEYNOTE-021 study. Lancet Oncology. 2016;**17**(11):1497-1508

[35] Davies M, Duffield EA. Safety of checkpoint inhibitors for cancer treatment: Strategies for patient monitoring and management of immune-mediated adverse events. ImmunoTargets and Therapy. 2017;**6**:51-71

[36] Chiang CL, Coukos G, Kandalaft LE. Whole tumor antigen vaccines: Where are we? Vaccines (Basel). 2015;**3**(2):344-372

[37] Heicappell R, Schirrmacher V, von Hoegen P, Ahlert T, Appelhans B. Prevention of metastatic spread by postoperative immunotherapy with virally modified autologous tumor cells. I. Parameters for optimal therapeutic effects. International Journal of Cancer. 1986;**37**(4):569-577

[38] Asada H, Kishida T, Hirai H, et al. Significant antitumor effects obtained by autologous tumor cell vaccine engineered to secrete interleukin (IL)-12 and IL-18 by means of the EBV/lipoplex. Molecular Therapy. 2002;**5**(5 Pt 1):609-616

[39] Mach N, Gillessen S, Wilson SB, Sheehan C, Mihm M, Dranoff G. Differences in dendritic cells stimulated in vivo by tumors engineered to secrete granulocyte-macrophage colony-stimulating factor or Flt3-ligand. Cancer Research. 2000;**60**(12):3239-3246

[40] Dranoff G. Targets of protective tumor immunity. Annals of the New York Academy of Sciences. 2009;**1174**:74-80

[41] Sondak VK, Sabel MS, Mule JJ. Allogeneic and autologous melanoma vaccines: Where have we been and where are we going? Clinical Cancer Research. 2006;**12**(7 Pt 2):2337s-2341s

[42] Small EJ, Sacks N, Nemunaitis J, et al. Granulocyte macrophage colony-stimulating factor--secreting allogeneic cellular immunotherapy for hormone-refractory prostate cancer. Clinical Cancer Research. 2007;**13**(13): 3883-3891

[43] Emens LA, Asquith JM, Leatherman JM, et al. Timed sequential treatment with cyclophosphamide, doxorubicin, and an allogeneic granulocyte-macrophage colony-stimulating factor-secreting breast tumor vaccine: A chemotherapy dose-ranging factorial study of safety and immune activation. Journal of Clinical Oncology. 2009;**27**(35):5911-5918

[44] Lutz E, Yeo CJ, Lillemoe KD, et al. A lethally irradiated allogeneic granulocyte-macrophage colony stimulating factor-secreting tumor vaccine for pancreatic adenocarcinoma. A phase II trial of safety, efficacy, and immune activation. Annals of Surgery. 2011;**253**(2):328-335

[45] van den Eertwegh AJ, Versluis J, van den Berg HP, et al. Combined immunotherapy with granulocyte-macrophage colony-stimulating factor-transduced allogeneic prostate cancer cells and ipilimumab in patients with metastatic castration-resistant prostate cancer: A phase 1 dose-escalation trial. The Lancet Oncology. 2012;**13**(5):509-517

[46] Nemunaitis J, Nemunaitis M, Senzer N, et al. Phase II trial of Belagenpumatucel-L, a TGF-beta2 antisense gene modified allogeneic tumor vaccine in advanced non small cell lung cancer (NSCLC) patients. Cancer Gene Therapy. 2009;**16**(8):620-624

[47] Banchereau J, Steinman RM. Dendritic cells and the control of immunity. Nature. 1998;**392**(6673):245-252

[48] Mildner A, Jung S. Development and function of dendritic cell subsets. Immunity. 2014;**40**(5):642-656

[49] Dudziak D, Kamphorst AO, Heidkamp GF, et al. Differential antigen processing by dendritic cell subsets in vivo. Science. 2007;**315**(5808):107-111

[50] Karachi A, Fazeli M, Karimi MH, et al. Evaluation of immunomodulatory effects of mesenchymal stem cells soluble factors on miR-155 and miR-23b expression in mice dendritic cells. Immunological Investigations. 2015;**44**(5):427-437

[51] Dastmalchi F, Karachi A, Azari H, Mitchell D, Rahman M. Strategy to enhance DC migration for increased efficacy of dendritic cells vaccine immunotherapy. Neuro-Oncology. 2017;**19**(suppl_6):vi125

[52] Frankenberger B, Schendel DJ. Third generation dendritic cell vaccines for tumor immunotherapy. European Journal of Cell Biology. 2012;**91**(1):53-58

[53] Dastmalchi F, Karachi A, Mitchell D, Rahman M. Dendritic Cell Therapy. In: eLS. Chichester: John Wiley & Sons, Ltd; 2018. DOI: 10.1002/9780470015902.a0024243

[54] Batich KA, Reap EA, Archer GE, et al. Long-term survival in glioblastoma with cytomegalovirus pp65-targeted vaccination. Clinical Cancer Research. 2017;**23**(8):1898-1909

[55] Nair SK, Morse M, Boczkowski D, et al. Induction of tumor-specific cytotoxic T lymphocytes in cancer patients by autologous tumor RNA-transfected dendritic cells. Annals of Surgery. 2002;**235**(4):540-549

[56] Murphy G, Tjoa B, Ragde H, Kenny G, Boynton A. Phase I clinical trial: T-cell therapy for prostate cancer using autologous dendritic cells pulsed with HLA-A0201-specific peptides from prostate-specific membrane antigen. The Prostate. 1996;**29**(6):371-380

[57] Schuler-Thurner B, Schultz ES, Berger TG, et al. Rapid induction of tumor-specific type 1 T helper cells in metastatic melanoma patients by vaccination with mature, cryopreserved, peptide-loaded monocyte-derived dendritic cells. The Journal of Experimental Medicine. 2002;**195**(10):1279-1288

[58] Rosenblatt J, Vasir B, Uhl L, et al. Vaccination with dendritic cell/tumor fusion cells results in cellular and humoral antitumor immune responses in patients with multiple myeloma. Blood. 2011;**117**(2):393-402

[59] Longo DL. New therapies for castration-resistant prostate cancer. The New England Journal of Medicine. 2010;**363**(5):479-481

[60] Bonehill A, Tuyaerts S, Van Nuffel AM, et al. Enhancing the T-cell stimulatory capacity of human dendritic cells by co-electroporation with CD40L, CD70 and constitutively active TLR4 encoding mRNA. Molecular Therapy. 2008;**16**(6):1170-1180

[61] Dannull J, Nair S, Su Z, et al. Enhancing the immunostimulatory function of dendritic cells by transfection with mRNA encoding OX40 ligand. Blood. 2005;**105**(8):3206-3213

[62] Grunebach F, Kayser K, Weck MM, Muller MR, Appel S, Brossart P. Cotransfection of dendritic cells with RNA coding for HER-2/neu and 4-1BBL increases the induction of tumor antigen specific cytotoxic T lymphocytes. Cancer Gene Therapy. 2005;**12**(9):749-756

[63] Tuyaerts S, Aerts JL, Corthals J, et al. Current approaches in dendritic cell generation and future implications for cancer immunotherapy. Cancer Immunology, Immunotherapy. 2007;**56**(10):1513-1537

[64] Iinuma H, Okinaga K, Fukushima R, et al. Superior

protective and therapeutic effects of IL-12 and IL-18 gene-transduced dendritic neuroblastoma fusion cells on liver metastasis of murine neuroblastoma. Journal of Immunology. 2006;**176**(6):3461-3469

[65] Kang TH, Bae HC, Kim SH, et al. Modification of dendritic cells with interferon-gamma-inducible protein-10 gene to enhance vaccine potency. The Journal of Gene Medicine. 2009;**11**(10):889-898

[66] Minkis K, Kavanagh DG, Alter G, et al. Type 2 bias of T cells expanded from the blood of melanoma patients switched to type 1 by IL-12p70 mRNA-transfected dendritic cells. Cancer Research. 2008;**68**(22):9441-9450

[67] Ogawa F, Iinuma H, Okinaga K. Dendritic cell vaccine therapy by immunization with fusion cells of interleukin-2 gene-transduced, spleen-derived dendritic cells and tumour cells. Scandinavian Journal of Immunology. 2004;**59**(5):432-439

[68] Okada N, Mori N, Koretomo R, et al. Augmentation of the migratory ability of DC-based vaccine into regional lymph nodes by efficient CCR7 gene transduction. Gene Therapy. 2005;**12**(2):129-139

[69] Song XT, Evel-Kabler K, Shen L, Rollins L, Huang XF, Chen SY. A20 is an antigen presentation attenuator, and its inhibition overcomes regulatory T cell-mediated suppression. Nature Medicine. 2008;**14**(3):258-265

[70] Palmer DC, Restifo NP. Suppressors of cytokine signaling (SOCS) in T cell differentiation, maturation, and function. Trends in Immunology. 2009;**30**(12):592-602

[71] Yu X, Yi H, Guo C, et al. Pattern recognition scavenger receptor CD204 attenuates Toll-like receptor 4-induced NF-kappaB activation by directly inhibiting ubiquitination of tumor necrosis factor (TNF) receptor-associated factor 6. The Journal of Biological Chemistry. 2011;**286**(21):18795-18806

[72] van der Bruggen P, Traversari C, Chomez P, et al. A gene encoding an antigen recognized by cytolytic T lymphocytes on a human melanoma. Science. 1991;**254**(5038):1643-1647

[73] De Smet C, Lurquin C, van der Bruggen P, De Plaen E, Brasseur F, Boon T. Sequence and expression pattern of the human MAGE2 gene. Immunogenetics. 1994;**39**(2):121-129

[74] Gnjatic S, Ritter E, Buchler MW, et al. Seromic profiling of ovarian and pancreatic cancer. Proceedings of the National Academy of Sciences of the United States of America. 2010;**107**(11):5088-5093

[75] Karbach J, Neumann A, Atmaca A, et al. Efficient in vivo priming by vaccination with recombinant NY-ESO-1 protein and CpG in antigen naive prostate cancer patients. Clinical Cancer Research. 2011;**17**(4): 861-870

[76] Correale P, Walmsley K, Nieroda C, et al. In vitro generation of human cytotoxic T lymphocytes specific for peptides derived from prostate-specific antigen. Journal of the National Cancer Institute. 1997;**89**(4):293-300

[77] Kantoff PW, Higano CS, Shore ND, et al. Sipuleucel-T immunotherapy for castration-resistant prostate cancer. The New England Journal of Medicine. 2010;**363**(5):411-422

[78] Bakker AB, Schreurs MW, de Boer AJ, et al. Melanocyte lineage-specific antigen gp100 is recognized by melanoma-derived tumor-infiltrating lymphocytes. The Journal of Experimental Medicine. 1994;**179**(3):1005-1009

[79] Kawakami Y, Eliyahu S, Sakaguchi K, et al. Identification of the immunodominant peptides of the MART-1 human melanoma antigen recognized by the majority of HLA-A2-restricted tumor infiltrating lymphocytes. The Journal of Experimental Medicine. 1994;**180**(1):347-352

[80] Parkhurst MR, Fitzgerald EB, Southwood S, Sette A, Rosenberg SA, Kawakami Y. Identification of a shared HLA-A*0201-restricted T-cell epitope from the melanoma antigen tyrosinase-related protein 2 (TRP2). Cancer Research. 1998;**58**(21):4895-4901

[81] Jaramillo A, Majumder K, Manna PP, et al. Identification of HLA-A3-restricted CD8+ T cell epitopes derived from mammaglobin-A, a tumor-associated antigen of human breast cancer. International Journal of Cancer. 2002;**102**(5):499-506

[82] Tsang KY, Zaremba S, Nieroda CA, Zhu MZ, Hamilton JM, Schlom J. Generation of human cytotoxic T cells specific for human carcinoembryonic antigen epitopes from patients immunized with recombinant vaccinia-CEA vaccine. Journal of the National Cancer Institute. 1995;**87**(13):982-990

[83] Finn OJ, Gantt KR, Lepisto AJ, Pejawar-Gaddy S, Xue J, Beatty PL. Importance of MUC1 and spontaneous mouse tumor models for understanding the immunobiology of human adenocarcinomas. Immunologic Research. 2011;**50**(2-3):261-268

[84] Disis ML, Wallace DR, Gooley TA, et al. Concurrent trastuzumab and HER2/neu-specific vaccination in patients with metastatic breast cancer. Journal of Clinical Oncology. 2009;**27**(28):4685-4692

[85] Schmollinger JC, Vonderheide RH, Hoar KM, et al. Melanoma inhibitor of apoptosis protein (ML-IAP) is a target for immune-mediated tumor destruction. Proceedings of the National Academy of Sciences of the United States of America. 2003;**100**(6):3398-3403

[86] Schmidt SM, Schag K, Muller MR, et al. Survivin is a shared tumor-associated antigen expressed in a broad variety of malignancies and recognized by specific cytotoxic T cells. Blood. 2003;**102**(2):571-576

[87] Kawai T, Akira S. Toll-like receptors and their crosstalk with other innate receptors in infection and immunity. Immunity. 2011;**34**(5):637-650

[88] Heldwein KA, Liang MD, Andresen TK, et al. TLR2 and TLR4 serve distinct roles in the host immune response against Mycobacterium bovis BCG. Journal of Leukocyte Biology. 2003;**74**(2):277-286

[89] Mata-Haro V, Cekic C, Martin M, Chilton PM, Casella CR, Mitchell TC. The vaccine adjuvant monophosphoryl lipid A as a TRIF-biased agonist of TLR4. Science. 2007;**316**(5831):1628-1632

[90] Clarke MA, Wentzensen N, Mirabello L, et al. Human papillomavirus DNA methylation as a potential biomarker for cervical cancer. Cancer Epidemiology, Biomarkers & Prevention. 2012;**21**(12): 2125-2137

[91] Kumai T, Kobayashi H, Harabuchi Y, Celis E. Peptide vaccines in cancer-old concept revisited. Current Opinion in Immunology. 2017;**45**:1-7

[92] Aurisicchio L, Ciliberto G. Genetic cancer vaccines: Current status and perspectives. Expert Opinion on Biological Therapy. 2012;**12**(8):1043-1058

[93] Liu MA. DNA vaccines: An historical perspective and view to

the future. Immunological Reviews. 2011;**239**(1):62-84

[94] Stratford R, Douce G, Zhang-Barber L, Fairweather N, Eskola J, Dougan G. Influence of codon usage on the immunogenicity of a DNA vaccine against tetanus. Vaccine. 2000;**19**(7-8):810-815

[95] Barber GN. Cytoplasmic DNA innate immune pathways. Immunological Reviews. 2011;**243**(1):99-108

[96] Yang B, Jeang J, Yang A, Wu TC, Hung CF. DNA vaccine for cancer immunotherapy. Human Vaccines & Immunotherapeutics. 2014;**10**(11):3153-3164

[97] Walter P, Johnson AE. Signal sequence recognition and protein targeting to the endoplasmic reticulum membrane. Annual Review of Cell Biology. 1994;**10**:87-119

[98] Rice J, Ottensmeier CH, Stevenson FK. DNA vaccines: Precision tools for activating effective immunity against cancer. Nature Reviews. Cancer. 2008;**8**(2):108-120

[99] Dharmapuri S, Aurisicchio L, Neuner P, Verdirame M, Ciliberto G, La Monica N. An oral TLR7 agonist is a potent adjuvant of DNA vaccination in transgenic mouse tumor models. Cancer Gene Therapy. 2009;**16**(5):462-472

[100] Orlandi F, Guevara-Patino JA, Merghoub T, Wolchok JD, Houghton AN, Gregor PD. Combination of epitope-optimized DNA vaccination and passive infusion of monoclonal antibody against HER2/neu leads to breast tumor regression in mice. Vaccine. 2011;**29**(20):3646-3654

[101] Fiedler K, Lazzaro S, Lutz J, Rauch S, Heidenreich R. mRNA cancer vaccines. Recent Results in Cancer Research. 2016;**209**:61-85

[102] Fotin-Mleczek M, Zanzinger K, Heidenreich R, et al. Highly potent mRNA based cancer vaccines represent an attractive platform for combination therapies supporting an improved therapeutic effect. The Journal of Gene Medicine. 2012;**14**(6):428-439

[103] Rosenberg SA, Restifo NP. Adoptive cell transfer as personalized immunotherapy for human cancer. Science. 2015;**348**(6230):62-68

[104] Verdegaal EM. Adoptive cell therapy: A highly successful individualized therapy for melanoma with great potential for other malignancies. Current Opinion in Immunology. 2016;**39**:90-95

[105] Yee C, Thompson JA, Byrd D, et al. Adoptive T cell therapy using antigen-specific CD8+ T cell clones for the treatment of patients with metastatic melanoma: in vivo persistence, migration, and antitumor effect of transferred T cells. Proceedings of the National Academy of Sciences of the United States of America. 2002;**99**(25):16168-16173

[106] Bryant KL, Mancias JD, Kimmelman AC, Der CJ. KRAS: Feeding pancreatic cancer proliferation. Trends in Biochemical Sciences. 2014;**39**(2):91-100

[107] Tran E, Robbins PF, Lu YC, et al. T-cell transfer therapy targeting mutant KRAS in cancer. The New England Journal of Medicine. 2016;**375**(23):2255-2262

[108] Morgan RA, Dudley ME, Wunderlich JR, et al. Cancer regression in patients after transfer of genetically engineered lymphocytes. Science. 2006;**314**(5796):126-129

[109] Robbins PF, Morgan RA, Feldman SA, et al. Tumor regression in patients with metastatic synovial cell sarcoma and melanoma using genetically engineered lymphocytes reactive with

NY-ESO-1. Journal of Clinical Oncology. 2011;**29**(7):917-924

[110] Donohue JH, Rosenstein M, Chang AE, Lotze MT, Robb RJ, Rosenberg SA. The systemic administration of purified interleukin 2 enhances the ability of sensitized murine lymphocytes to cure a disseminated syngeneic lymphoma. Journal of Immunology. 1984;**132**(4):2123-2128

[111] Dastmalchi F, Karachi A, Allison JR, Basso K, Mitchell D, Rahman M. In vivo cellular tracking with 13C labeling of adopetive transferred T cells for the treatment of brain tumors. Neuro-Oncology. 2017;**19**(suppl_6):vi119

[112] Leone P, Shin EC, Perosa F, Vacca A, Dammacco F, Racanelli V. MHC class I antigen processing and presenting machinery: Organization, function, and defects in tumor cells. Journal of the National Cancer Institute. 2013;**105**(16):1172-1187

[113] Brudno JN, Somerville RP, Shi V, et al. Allogeneic T cells that express an anti-CD19 chimeric antigen receptor induce remissions of B-cell malignancies that Progress after allogeneic hematopoietic stem-cell transplantation without causing graft-versus-host disease. Journal of Clinical Oncology. 2016;**34**(10):1112-1121

[114] Kochenderfer JN, Dudley ME, Kassim SH, et al. Chemotherapy-refractory diffuse large B-cell lymphoma and indolent B-cell malignancies can be effectively treated with autologous T cells expressing an anti-CD19 chimeric antigen receptor. Journal of Clinical Oncology. 2015;**33**(6):540-549

[115] Maude SL, Frey N, Shaw PA, et al. Chimeric antigen receptor T cells for sustained remissions in leukemia. The New England Journal of Medicine. 2014;**371**(16):1507-1517

[116] Porter DL, Levine BL, Kalos M, Bagg A, June CH. Chimeric antigen receptor-modified T cells in chronic lymphoid Leukemia; chimeric antigen receptor-modified T cells for acute lymphoid Leukemia; chimeric antigen receptor T cells for sustained remissions in Leukemia. The New England Journal of Medicine. 2016;**374**(10):998

[117] Ninomiya S, Narala N, Huye L, et al. Tumor indoleamine 2,3-dioxygenase (IDO) inhibits CD19-CAR T cells and is downregulated by lymphodepleting drugs. Blood. 2015;**125**(25):3905-3916

[118] Kakimi K, Karasaki T, Matsushita H, Sugie T. Advances in personalized cancer immunotherapy. Breast Cancer. 2017;**24**:16-24

Section 2

Digestive Cancers

Chapter 3

Advances in the Treatment of Pancreatic Cancer

Michelle Marie Fillion

Abstract

Pancreatic cancer is an aggressive solid organ malignancy with a high mortality rate. There has only been significant improvement in the overall survival until the last 5–10 years. The current trend toward the neoadjuvant approach of pancreatic cancer has shown success in tumor response, resection rate, and even overall survival. Using dedicated pancreatic protocol cross-sectional imaging, one can now follow the tumor and pancreatic parenchyma interface as well as tumor markers to predict treatment response. Aggressive combination chemotherapy regimens such as FOLFIRINOX (5-fluorouracil, leucovorin, oxaliplatin, and irinotecan), appropriate patient selection, and multidisciplinary treatment teams have made an impact in the current management of pancreatic cancer. Surgical intervention is still the mainstay treatment of pancreatic cancer. The role of routine radiation therapy is still unknown but may benefit in situations with positive margins.

Keywords: pancreatic cancer, neoadjuvant chemotherapy, FOLFIRINOX

1. Introduction

1.1 Incidence and mortality

Pancreatic cancer is the 13th most common malignancy worldwide, which was diagnosed in approximately 338,000 people in 2012. Pancreatic cancer is a very aggressive form of malignancy resulting in the seventh leading cause of cancer deaths worldwide, over 331,000 deaths in 2012 alone. The worldwide incidence of new pancreatic cancers was 4.9 in 100,000 persons with an associated mortality rate of approximately 4%. The incidence and deaths of pancreatic cancer is higher in developed countries, 188,000 and 184,000 persons as compared to less developed regions, 150,000 and 146,000 persons [1].

Specifically looking at the USA, pancreatic cancer is the eighth most common type of malignancy and the fourth leading cause of cancer deaths. There are estimated 55,440 new cases of pancreatic cancer that will be diagnosed in the USA in 2018 and result in estimated 44,330 deaths. Incidence rate of pancreatic cancer has increased 1% per year from 2005 to 2014 [2].

Most pancreatic cancers develop from the pancreatic exocrine tissue (94%), such as invasive ductal adenocarcinoma, while the remaining 6% of tumors stem from the hormone-producing islet cells, such as insulinomas, gastrinomas, and other pancreatic neuroendocrine tumors (pNETs). Those pNets will typically occur in younger patients with a better overall prognosis. The focus of this chapter will be on invasive pancreatic ductal adenocarcinoma [2].

The overall pancreatic cancer mortality rate has shown only slight improvement over the past 35 years. In 1975, pancreatic cancer mortality rate was observed at 3.1%, and in 2000, it increased to 5.2%. The largest incremental improvement in pancreatic cancer survival has occurred over the past 10 years (2008–2104), with the all stage 5 year survival between 8 and 8.5% [2–4].

For the small percentage of patients with early-stage localized pancreatic cancer (10%), the 5-year survival is between 32 and 34.3%. Once regional lymph node involvement has developed, the 5 year survival decreases to 11.5–12%. Unfortunately, most pancreatic cancer patients (52%) are diagnosed with distant metastatic disease, and that 5-year survival is only 3% [2, 3].

1.2 Risk factors

At this point in the time, the cause of pancreatic cancer is still unknown. Increasing age is a significant risk factor for developing pancreatic cancer. The median age of diagnosis of pancreatic cancer in both sexes is at 70 years old. In addition, men have an increased incidence of developing pancreatic cancer as compared to women, 14.4 vs. 11.2 per 100,000 persons across all race and ethnicity [1–3].

There have been several risk factors to develop pancreatic cancer associated with race/ethnicity, environmental, dietary, medical, and genetic exposures identified (**Table 1**). Race is also another significant risk factor. African-Americans have the highest incidence (9.9 per 100,000 persons) and mortality (9.4 per 100,000 persons) of pancreatic cancer as compared to non-African-Americans [4]. In addition, Jews of Ashkenazi heritage also have an increased incidence of pancreatic cancer. The age standardized incidence rate of pancreatic cancer for Israeli Jews (7.2 per 100,000 males and 5.7 per 100,000 females) exceeds the incidence of Israeli non-Jews (4.0 per 100,000 males and 2.9 per 100,000 females) [5].

There are also several hereditary conditions associated with increased risk for pancreatic cancer (**Table 2**). While persons with these genetic syndromes are at increased risk for pancreatic cancer, they only account for 5% of all pancreatic diagnoses. Familial cases of pancreatic cancer are at increased incidence to develop secondary primary cancers as compared to non-familial-based cancers. Of those listed, Peutz-Jeghers and hereditary pancreatitis syndromes have the highest risk of developing pancreatic cancer [6–12].

Environmental	Race	Medical	Dietary
Cigarette smoking Second-hand smoke Alcohol Asbestos Pesticides Herbicides Residential Radon Coal Products Welding Products Radiation	African-American Ashkenazi Jews	Pancreatitis Diabetes *Helicobacter pylori* infection Cirrhosis	High saturated fat diet Nitrosamines Overweight Obesity

Table 1.
Risk factors for developing pancreatic cancer.

Genetic Syndrome	Gene Mutation	Relative Risk
Hereditary Pancreatitis	PRSS1 (7q35)	50-80 times
Hereditary Nonpolyposis Colorectal Cancer (HNPCC, Lynch Syndrome)	hMSH2; hMLH1; hPMS2; hMSH6	Not defined
Hereditary Breast and Ovarian Cancer Syndrome (HBOC)	BRCA2 (13q12)	10 times
Familial Adenomatous Polyposis (FAP)	APC (5q21)	5 times
Familial Atypical Multiple Mole Melanoma (FAMMM) Syndrome	P16(9p21)	20-34 times
Peutz-Jeghers Syndrome	STK11/LKB1 (19p13)	132 times
Ataxia-telangiectasia	ATM (11q22-23)	Not defined

Table 2.
Genetic syndromes with increased risk of pancreatic cancer.

Tobacco use is the most well-established modifiable risk factor for developing pancreatic cancer and accounts for up to 30% of all pancreatic cancer cases. There is at least a twofold increase in risk for developing pancreatic cancer in cigarette smoker than a non-smoker. The risk also increases with an increase in the number of cigarettes and duration of smoking. It may take up to 20 years after cessation of cigarette smoking for one's risk of pancreatic cancer to be equal to take of a non-smoker [13].

2. Treatment of resectable disease

2.1 Imaging considerations

The current standard in pancreatic cancer staging is by use of a 64-slice multidetector computed tomography (CT). Specific CT pancreatic protocols can accurately stage the cancer and assess for resectability. These protocols include both the use of low-density oral contrast and nonionic iodinated contrast and scanned 30–45 seconds then again 60 seconds after injection to capture both arterial and venous phases. The arterial phase will allow for good visualization of the celiac axis, common hepatic artery, superior mesenteric artery, and gastroduodenal artery. The venous phase will show enhanced visualization of the portal vein, superior mesenteric vein, splenic vein, pancreatic parenchyma, and the liver to assess for metastatic disease [14, 15].

2.2 Surgical considerations

Only 20% of patients who present with pancreatic cancer can undergo surgical resection since most patients present with either unresectable or metastatic disease. The only chance for a curative treatment is with the inclusion of successful surgical removal of the cancer. To determine the patient's eligibility for pancreatic resection, an experienced pancreatic surgeon is required to review the dedicated pancreatic cross-sectional imaging. The relationship of the tumor to the major intra-abdominal vessels determines the resectability of the pancreatic cancer. Decisions regarding diagnostic and management and resectability should involve multidisciplinary consultation at high-volume center, at least 15–20 pancreatic resections per year [14].

In 2006, the National Comprehensive Cancer Network (NCCN) criteria initially defined pancreatic cancers resectability status into three classifications: resectable, borderline resectable, and unresectable. Since that time, there have been several varying definitions of tumor resectability that have evolved over the past decade. Several international surgical societies such as the American Hepato-Pancreatico-Biliary Association (AHPBA), Society of Surgical Oncology (SSO), Society for Surgery of the Alimentary Tract (SSAT), and International Association of Pancreatology (IAP) have issued consensus statements on the definition and criteria of resectability and borderline resectable pancreatic cancers as illustrated in **Table 3** [14–16].

For a tumor to be considered resectable, it must not be in contact with the portal vein (PV) or superior mesenteric vein (SMV) per AHPBA/SSO/SSAT and IAP or less than 180° of contact with SMV/PV by NCCN criteria. By meeting these criteria, the surgeon believes there is a high likelihood of removing the cancer without leaving behind any residual tumor (R0 resection). When pancreatic cancers are classified as borderline resectable based on the vascular involvement, it means that there is a higher likelihood of having residual microscopic disease (R1 resection) if one was to proceed with upfront surgery. Borderline resectable means just that it is not quite resectable but not completely unresectable either. The criteria are less than 180° of arterial involvement of the superior mesenteric artery (SMA) or common hepatic artery (CHA) of celiac axis (CA). It also means there can be greater than 180° of involvement of SMV or even complete encasement of SMV or PV but still suitable for resection vascular reconstruction. Unresectable disease has greater than 180° of arterial involvement of SMA, CHA, or CA or non-reconstructable vein involvement including the first jejunal branch [14–16].

The best outcomes come from margin negative surgical resection with no residual microscopic disease (R0). There is current debate at the true definition of R1 resection as either no microscopic tumor cells at the resection margin or if tumor cells are less than 1 mm from the resection margin. It has been found that the 5-year survival rate has been improved in patients with greater than 1 mm of clearance as compared to those with less than 1 mm. Margins with 0 mm, less than 1 mm, or greater than 1 mm had 5-year survival rates at 16.3, 12.4, and 27.6%, respectively [17]. There is no benefit to performing a surgical resection if gross tumor (R2 resection) will be the result as the prognosis is similar to patients with non-operative management [18].

	NCCN	AHPBA/ SSO/ SSAT	IAP
Resectable Vein Artery	No tumor contact with SMV and PV or <180° contact without vein contour irregularity	No SMV and PV abutment, distortion, tumor thrombus or venous encasement	No tumor contact or narrowing to SMV or PV
	No artery tumor contact of CA, SMA, or CHA	Clear fat planes around CA, SMA and CHA	No tumor contact to SMA, CA, CHA
Borderline Resectable Vein Artery	Tumor contact of SMV/PV > 180° or contact <180° resulting in vein irregularity or thrombus but with suitable proximal and distal vessel for safe resection and reconstruction Tumor contact to inferior vena cava	Abutment with or without impingement of SMV or PV lumen, short segment occlusion or encasement but with suitable vessel distal and proximal to allow for safe resection and reconstruction	Tumor contact >180° without deformity of SMV or PV
	Head/Uncinate: Contact CHA without extension to CA Tumor contact <180° of SMA Tumor contact with variant anatomy Tumor contact <180° CA **Body/Tail:** Tumor contact with CA >180° w/o involvement of aorta and intact GDA	GDA encasement w either short encasement of direct abutment of CHA without extension to CA Tumor abutment of SMA not to exceed 180° degrees circumference of vessel wall	Tumor contact < 180° without deformity/stenosis of SMA, CA, CHA
Unresectable Vein Artery	Unreconstructible SMV/PV due to tumor involvement or occlusion Contact with first jejunal branch into SMV		Bilateral narrowing/ occlusion beyond inferior border of duodenum
	Head/Uncinate: Tumor contact w SMA >180° Tumor contact with CA. 180° **Body/Tail:** Tumor contact >180° SMA or CA Tumor contact with CHA >180°		Tumor contact or invasion of the aorta

Table 3.
Definitions and criteria of resectable, borderline resectable and unresectable pancreatic cancer.

Pancreatic surgery should involve high-volume surgeons with the expertise in pancreatic resection. Decisions regarding the management of pancreatic cancer patients require a multidisciplinary team. The location of the tumor and extent of disease will dictate the surgical approaches. Pancreatic head and uncinate tumors require pancreaticoduodenectomy (Whipple procedure) with reconstruction of the pancreas, bile duct, and stomach. If possible, the aim is to preserve the pylorus to limit bile acid reflux and gastric emptying. Tumors that exist in the body and tail of the pancreas will typically require a left-sided surgical resection, distal pancreatectomy, and splenectomy. Borderline resectable and locally advanced cancers may also require venous and/or arterial reconstruction at the time of surgical resection of the pancreatic cancer.

2.3 Chemotherapy

In patients with pancreatic cancer, the overall survival has improved due to systemic chemotherapy and combination therapies. It is still standard treatment to perform upfront surgical resection for resectable pancreatic cancer followed by adjuvant chemotherapy. However, there has been a shift toward upfront neoadjuvant chemotherapy in order to select out patients with latent metastatic disease or to downstage borderline and locally advanced cancers.

The ESPAC-1 (European Study Group for Pancreatic Cancer) showed that there was improvement in overall survival using surgery plus adjuvant 5-fluorouracil (5-FU) plus folinic acid (FA). This three-tracked trial compared patients treated with chemotherapy alone, surgical resection alone, or chemotherapy plus radiation therapy. The highest 5-year survival was seen in the chemotherapy arm 21% as compared to surgery alone 8% and chemoradiation 11%. This revealed the only significant survival benefit was with adjuvant chemotherapy [19].

The Charite Onkologie study (CONKO-001) from 2007 compared adjuvant gemcitabine therapy to observation in patients undergoing surgical resection of pancreatic cancer. In the treatment arm, patients received 6 cycles of adjuvant gemcitabine. Patients treated with adjuvant gemcitabine vs. surgery alone had statistically significant increased median overall survival of 22.8 months and 5-year survival of 21% compared to 20.2 months and 5-year survival of 9%. Gemcitabine also significantly delayed the development of recurrent disease as compared to observation alone [20].

The ESPAC-3 was a large randomized controlled trial which compared adjuvant 5-FU plus leucovorin or gemcitabine in patients who underwent RO or R1 resection of pancreatic cancer. This was initially a three-arm study comparing 5-FU plus leucovorin, gemcitabine, and observation; however, once the results of the ESPAC-1 were available, the observation arm was closed. Results of ESPAC-1, ESPAC-1 plus, and ESPAC-3 in subset analysis of 5-FU/FA vs. observation confirmed that adjuvant 5-FU/FA had superior overall survival as compared to observation after surgical resection. The 5 year survival for 5-FU/FA was 24% compared to observation which was 14% [21].

ESPAC-3 has enrolled 1088 patients and they were followed for over 6.5 years. Median survival for gemcitabine arm was 23.6 months while 5FU/leucovorin arm was 23 months [22]. This had shown that adjuvant gemcitabine had similar survival but less toxicity as compared to 5FU. At this point, there were now two different adjuvant treatment options for resected pancreatic cancer.

Van Hoof et al. (2013) performed a phase III trial in which metastatic pancreatic cancer patients were randomized to treatment with either nab-paclitaxel (125 mg per square meter of body surface area) plus gemcitabine (1000 mg per square meter) on days 1, 8, and 15 every 4 weeks or gemcitabine monotherapy

(1000 mg per square meter) weekly for 7 of 8 weeks and then on days 1, 8, and 15 every 4 weeks. The overall survival in the nab-paclitaxel-gemcitabine was 8.5 months as compared to gemcitabine alone with 6.7 months ($p > 0.001$). This doublet therapy did result in higher rates of myelosuppression and peripheral neuropathy than gemcitabine alone [23]. While this study was based on patients with metastatic disease, it advanced the adjuvant combined chemotherapy regimen in resected pancreatic cancer.

The ESPAC-4 went on to compare adjuvant gemcitabine and capecitabine with gemcitabine monotherapy in patients with resected pancreatic cancer. Capecitabine is an orally active fluoropyrimidine carbamate which can provide prolonged fluorouracil exposure at lower peak concentrations. The 5-year overall survival with gemcitabine and capecitabine compared to gemcitabine alone was 29% vs. 16% [24]. The new standard of care quickly adopted doublet therapy as the new standard of care.

The use of adjuvant FOLFIRINOX [fluorouracil (5-FU), leucovorin, irinotecan, oxaliplatin] has been extrapolated from the treatment of pancreatic cancer in the metastatic setting. In the ACCORD-11 trial, FOLFIRINOX was found to have a superior survival advantage over gemcitabine in metastatic pancreatic patients with median overall survival of 11.1 months vs. 6.8 months [25]. This study ultimately launched FOLFIRINOX into new treatment paradigms in the adjuvant and neoadjuvant settings.

The phase III PRODIGE 24/CCTG PA.6 trial compared a modified FOLFIRINOX regimen against single-agent gemcitabine therapy, as the results of the ESPAC-4 were not known at study design. This study used a modified FOLFIRINOX regimen: oxaliplatin 85 mg/m^2, leucovorin 400 mg/m^2, and irinotecan 180 mg/m^2 (dose reduced to 150 mg/m^2 after patient 162) on day 1 and continuous fluorouracil infusion 2.4 gm/m^2 over 46 hours. This regimen was repeated every 2 weeks for 12 cycles. The gemcitabine regimen was 1000 mg/m^2 once per 3 of 4 weeks for 6 cycles [26]. The response rate was 31.18% in the mFOLFIRINOX group and 11.3% in the gemcitabine group. The disease-free survival (DFS) and overall survival (OS) in the mFOLFIRINOX arm were 21.6 and 54.4 months, while the gemcitabine arm were 17.7 and 35.0 months repetitively. Grade 3 or 4 adverse events (neutropenia, diarrhea, neuropathy) were significantly higher in the FOLFIRINOX treatment arm than the gemcitabine arm [26].

mFOLFIRINOX has been the largest advancement in overall survival for resected pancreatic cancer patients, which more than doubled the previous median overall survival.

2.4 Radiation therapy

There are mixed opinions regarding the routine use of radiation therapy in pancreatic cancer. The ESPAC-1 did not reveal any significant survival benefit with chemoradiation [19]. A meta-analysis of five randomized controlled trials using adjuvant chemoradiation in patients who underwent curation resection was performed to assess the survival benefit. It appeared that adjuvant chemoradiation had benefitted the subset of patients with a positive margin status; however, it was not statistically significant [27].

The RTOG study looks to determine if the addition of gemcitabine to adjuvant fluorouracil chemoradiation improved survival as compared with fluorouracil. Patients were given either fluorouracil (continuous infusion 250 mg/m^2 per day) or 30 minutes infusion of gemcitabine (1000 mg/m^2 once a week) for 3 weeks prior to fluorouracil chemoradiation and for 12 weeks following chemoradiation. The median survival for the gemcitabine group was 20.5 months, while the median survival for the fluorouracil group was 16.9 months. There appeared to be a survival benefit, but it was not statistically significant [28].

The LAP07 randomized clinical trial aimed to assess if chemoradiation would improve overall survival after 4 months of gemcitabine and to assess erlotinib's effect on survival as well as in patients with locally advanced pancreatic cancer. There was no difference in overall survival between the chemotherapy alone vs. the addition of chemoradiation, 16.5 months vs. 15.2 months [29].

While variations may occur at different institutions, a common approach for resectable pancreatic cancer would include the surgical resection of the cancer followed by adjuvant chemotherapy. The use of radiation may be used in the adjuvant setting for positive margins following chemotherapy after proving no metastatic disease developed.

3. Treatment of borderline and locally advanced disease

3.1 Neoadjuvant therapy

For patients that present with borderline resectable and locally advanced pancreatic cancer, neoadjuvant chemotherapy with or without chemoradiation allows for systemic control and may improve the likelihood of a R0 resection. The initial rationale for upfront therapies is to potentially downstage tumors to become resectable with a higher R0 resection rate and to allow potential latent metastatic disease to declare itself. In addition, the use of neoadjuvant chemoradiation may be used to "sterilize" the tumor margins near vessel involvement. This allows for selection of the most appropriate patients who have the highest likelihood of long-term survival.

Based on the ACCORD-11 trial showing superior response to FOLFIRINOX, this regimen has now been used effectively in the neoadjuvant setting for borderline and locally advanced pancreatic cancers. Several series have been published showing institutional success. The Massachusetts General Hospital reported that patients treated with mFOLFIRINOX have significantly smaller tumors and lower rates of lymphovascular invasion and perineural invasion. The R0 resection was 92% [30]. Similar reports from the Ohio State University were also noted. They were also able to convert locally advanced and unresectable pancreatic cancers to resectable in 51% of patients who underwent neoadjuvant mFOLFIRINOX with R0 resection of 86% [31].

While patients are undergoing neoadjuvant chemotherapy, serial imaging with pancreatic protocol CT is used to observe for treatment response. In those patients that develop metastatic disease or progression to unresectable disease while undergoing neoadjuvant, their poor biology of disease had declared itself, and they were spared the major morbidity of a surgical resection. For those demonstrating stable or treatment response, the radiologic imaging can be used to predict treatment response. The appearance of the tumor and pancreatic parenchyma interface that becomes more distinct indicates a cytotoxic response which ultimately translates to pathologic response. The ideal response is for the tumor to pull away from the vessels and no longer see haziness around the vessels, which may indicate an infiltrative process. Another prognostic marker of treatment response is normalization of CA 19–9 during neoadjuvant therapy [32].

A pathologic complete response (pCR) can be found in approximately 10% of patients treated in the neoadjuvant approach with FOLFIRINOX and chemoradiation. This is also an independent prognostic risk factor for improved overall and disease-free survival [33]. Additionally, small tumor size, negative margins, and negative lymph node metastasis are favorable prognostic indicators for improved overall and disease-free survival.

The consensus for treatment of borderline resectable pancreatic cancer favors the neoadjuvant approach; however, it may vary per institution. After a multidisciplinary review at our hospital, the typical functional patient would undergo neoadjuvant chemotherapy (FOLFIRINOX) for 3–4 cycles followed by restaging with CT and CA 19–9. If stable or responding disease, then the patient would continue additional 3–4 cycles of FOLFIRINOX. The patient would again be restaged with CT and CA 19–9. Barring no metastatic disease developed and there was treatment response, the patient would then undergo surgical intervention. However, if the surgical margins were still threatened and there was concern for R1 resection, then the patient may undergo chemoradiation to "sterilize" the margins. Approximately 4–6 weeks after chemoradiation, the patient would ultimately undergo surgical resection.

4. Unresectable pancreatic cancer

Unresectable pancreatic cancer means that the tumor cannot safely be removed due to vascular involvement or metastatic disease. Patients may undergo aggressive chemotherapy with FOLFIRINOX, and a few may be able to convert to a resectable cancer. It is of utmost importance for early palliative care interventions in these patients. For those with biliary obstruction, the use of endoscopic biliary stents and percutaneous biliary drains may provide relief from the jaundice. If the tumor is found to be unresectable in the operating room, then palliative hepaticojejunostomy may be performed. Gastric outlet obstruction may also be relieved with endoscopically placed luminal stents. Additionally, surgical bypass may be performed in laparoscopic or open fashion with a gastrojejunostomy.

Pain can also become quite debilitating in patients with locally advanced unresectable pancreatic cancer. Celiac plexus neurolysis can be performed at the time of surgical exploration, or it may be performed by endoscopic or percutaneous routes.

Irreversible electroporation (IRE) is a nonthermal ablative modality which relies on high voltage (maximum 3,000 volts) small microsecond pulse lengths. This is a novel option typically used in locally advanced pancreatic adenocarcinoma of the head or neck that is not amendable to resection. Some institutions are now using IRE to assist with the resection of locally advanced tumors, but this is not standard at this time. The procedure may be performed open or percutaneously. Patients will typical undergo several months of neoadjuvant chemotherapy to not miss occult metastatic disease prior to IRE. IRE can improve progression-free survival from 6 to 14 months and overall survival from 23 to 20 months [34].

5. Clinical trials

There are several active clinical trials investigating additional treatment options for pancreatic cancer. Several phase II trials are looking at the use of targeted agents in addition to systemic chemotherapy. One study is evaluating the safety of niraparib, PARP [poly (ADP-ribose) polymerase] inhibitor, in advanced pancreatic cancer patients [35]. Another clinical trial at the Massachusetts General Hospital is using the checkpoint inhibitor, nivolumab, as programed death-1 (PD-1) inhibition in combination with losartan, FOLFIRINOX, stereotactic body radiation therapy (SBRT), and surgery in advanced pancreatic cancer. This is a three-armed study:

Arm 1 with FOLFIRINOX, SBRT, and then surgery; Arm 2 with FOLFIRINOX plus losartan, SBRT plus losartan, and then surgery; and Arm 3 with FOLFIRINOX plus losartan, SBRT plus nivolumab and losartan, and then surgery [36].

Reviewing the past studies on chemoradiation, one must keep in mind these studies were using monotherapy chemotherapy and conventional fractionated radiation therapy. There are now several clinical trials assessing the role of radiation therapy, specifically SBRT in the setting of FOLFIRINOX. SBRT utilizes high doses of ablative radiotherapy in typically 1–5 fractions.

The ALLIANCE A021501 is a randomized controlled trial using modified FOLFIRINOX regimen (oxaliplatin 85 mg/m^2, irinotecan 180 mg/m^2, leucovorin 400 mg/m^2, and infusional 5-fluorouracil 2400 mg/m^2 over 2 days for 4 cycles) in borderline resectable pancreatic head adenocarcinomas. Arm 1 is delivering this regimen for 8 cycles, while Arm 2 is receiving 7 cycles followed by SBRT (33–40 Gy in 5 fractions). The patient then undergoes pancreaticoduodenectomy followed 4 cycles of adjuvant-modified FOLFOX6 (oxaliplatin 85 mg/m^2, leucovorin 400 mg/m^2, bolus 5-fluorouracil 400 mg/m^2, and infusional 5-fluorouracil 2400 mg/m^2 over 2 days for 4 cycles). The main aim of this study is to assess 18-month overall survival, R0 resection, and event-free survival [37].

Another randomized controlled trial by the Pancreatic Cancer Radiotherapy Study Group (PanCRS) is assessing the progression-free survival between mFOLFIRINOX alone vs. mFOLFIRINOX and SBRT in locally advanced unresectable pancreatic cancer [38].

Also, a novel class of drug, cancer stemness inhibitors, is being investigated as a potential new treatment for pancreatic cancer. Napabucasin is an oral small molecule that blocks stem cell activity by targeting the signal transducer and activator of transcription 3 pathway. This pathway is believed to be an important pathway in the propagation of stem-cell-mediated cancer cells [39].

6. Conclusion

While pancreatic cancer is still an aggressive malignancy which is often lethal, there have been significant improvements in the systemic chemotherapy which has improved patients' overall survival. In addition, the radiographic quality has improved thus we are better able to appropriately stage patients for resectability from the onset. Future research in the use of targeted and immunotherapy and the promise of SBRT may control to improve the outcomes of pancreatic cancer patients. With the use of multidisciplinary treatment teams, aggressive combination chemotherapies and surgical resections, there is hope for the patients with pancreatic cancer.

Conflict of interest

The authors declare that there are no conflicts of interest.

DOI: http://dx.doi.org/10.5772/intechopen.82074

Author details

Michelle Marie Fillion
New Hanover Regional Medical Center, Wilmington, North Carolina, USA

*Address all correspondence to: michelle.fillion@nhrmc.org

References

[1] GLOBOCAN 2012: Estimated Cancer Incidence, Mortality and Prevalence worldwide in 2012. Available from: http://globocan.iarc.fr/Pages/fact_sheets_population.aspx

[2] Siegel RL, Miller KD, Jemal A. Cancer Statistics. CA: A Cancer Journal for Clinicians. 2018;**68**(1):7-30

[3] Noone AM, Howlader N, Krapcho M, et al. SEER Cancer Statistics Review, 1975–2015. Bethesda, MD: National Cancer Institute; 2018. Available from: https://seer.cancer.gov/csr/1975_2015/, based on November 2017 SEER data submission, posted to the SEER web site

[4] Saad AM, Turk T, Al-Husseini MJ, et al. Trends in pancreatic adenocarcinoma incidence and mortality in the United States in the last four decades: A SEER-based study. BMC Cancer. 2018;**18**:688-698

[5] Lynch HT, Deters CA, Lynch JF, et al. Familial pancreatic carcinoma in Jews. Familial Cancer. 2004;**3**:233-240

[6] Lowenfels AB, Maisonneuve P, Whitcomb DC, et al. Risk factors for cancer in hereditary pancreatitis. The Medical Clinics of North America. 2000; **84**:565-573

[7] Lynch HT, Voorhees GJ, Lanspa SJ, et al. Pancreatic carcinoma and hereditary nonpolyposis colorectal cancer: A family study. British Journal of Cancer. 1985;**52**:271-273

[8] Goggins M, Schutte M, Lu J, et al. Germline BRCA2 gene mutations in patients with apparently sporadic pancreatic carcinomas. Cancer Research. 1996;**56**:5360-5364

[9] Lynch HT, Smyrk T, Kern SE, et al. Familial pancreatic cancer: A review. Seminars in Oncology. 1996;**23**:251-275

[10] Lynch HT, Fusaro RM. Pancreatic cancer and the familial atypical multiple mole melanoma (FAMMM) syndrome. Pancreas. 1991;**6**:127-131

[11] Giardiello FM, Welsh SB, Hamilton SR, et al. Increased risk of cancer in the Peutz–Jeghers syndrome. The New England Journal of Medicine. 1987;**316**: 1511-1514

[12] Lynch HT, Brand RE, Deters CA, et al. Hereditary pancreatic cancer. Pancreatology. 2001;**1**:466-471

[13] Bosetti C, Lucenteforte E, Silverman DT, et al. Cigarette smoking and pancreatic cancer: An analysis from the International Pancreatic Cancer Case-Control Consortium (PancC4). Annals of Oncology. 2012;**23**(7):1880-1888

[14] Callery MP, Change KJ, Fishman EK, et al. Pretreatment assessment of resectable and borderline resectable pancreatic cancer: Expert consensus statement. Annals of Surgical Oncology. 2009;**16**:1727-1733

[15] National Comprehensive Cancer Network: NCCN Guidelines: Pancreatic Adenocarcinoma 2. 2018. Criteria for defining resectability status. Available from: https://www.nccn.org/professionals/physician_gls/pdf/pancreatic.pdf

[16] Isaji S, Mizunoa S, Windsor JA, et al. International consensus on definition and criteria of borderline resectable pancreatic ductal adenocarcinoma 2017. Pancreatology. 2018;**18**:2-11

[17] Van Roessel S, Kasumova GG, Tabatabaie O, et al. Pathological margin clearance and survival after pancreaticoduodenectomy in a US and European Pancreatic Center. Annals of Surgical Oncology. 2018;**25**:1760-1767

[18] Lopez NE, Prendergast C, Lowy AM. Borderline resectable pancreatic cancer: Definitions and management. World Journal of Gastroenterology. 2014;**20**(31):10740-10751

[19] Neoptolemos JP, Dunn JA, Moffitt DD, et al. ESPAC-1: A European, randomized controlled trial of chemoradiotherapy and chemotherapy after resection of pancreatic cancer. The New England Journal of Medicine. 2004;**350**:1200-1210

[20] Oettle H, Post S, Neuhaus P, et al. Adjuvant chemotherapy with gemcitabine vs observation in patient undergoing curative intent resection of pancreatic cancer: A randomized controlled trial. JAMA. 2007;**297**(3): 267-277

[21] Neoptolemos JP, Stocken DD, Smith c T, et al. Adjuvant 5-fluorouracil and folinic acid vs observation for pancreatic cancer: Composite data from the ESPAC-1 and -3(v1) trials. British Journal of Cancer. 2009;**100**(2): 246-250

[22] Neopltolemos JP, Stocken DD, Bassi C, et al. Adjuvant chemotherapy with fluorouracil plus folinic acid vs gemcitabine following pancreatic cancer resection: A randomized controlled trial. JAMA. 2010;**304**(10):1073-1081

[23] Von Hoff DD, Ervin T, Arena FP, et al. Increased survival in pancreatic cancer with nab-paclitaxel plus gemcitabine. The New England Journal of Medicine. 2013;**369**: 1691-1703

[24] Neoptolemos JP, Palmer DH, Ghaneh EF, et al. Comparison of adjuvant gemcitabine and capecitabine with gemcitabine monotherapy in patients with resected pancreatic cancer (ESPAC-4): A multicenter, open label randomized, phase 3 trial. Lancet. 2017; **389**:1011-1024

[25] Conroy T, Desseigne F, Ychou M, et al. FOLFIRINOX vs gemcitabine for metastatic pancreatic cancer. The New England Journal of Medicine. 2011;**364**: 1817-1825

[26] Conroy T. PRODIGE 24: Comparing adjuvant chemotherapy with gemcitabine versus mfolfirinox to treat resected pancreatic adenocarcinoma. In: ASCO Annual Meeting; Chicago, IL, USA. 2018

[27] Stocken DD, Buechler MW, Dervenis C, et al. Meta-analysis of randomised adjuvant therapy trials for pancreatic cancer. British Journal of Cancer. 2005;**92**(8):1372-1381

[28] Regine WF, Winter KA, Abrams RA, et al. Fluorouracil vs gemcitabine chemotherapy before and after fluorouracil-based chemoradiation following resection of pancreatic adenocarcinoma: A randomized controlled trial. JAMA. 2008;**299**(9): 1019-1026

[29] Hammel P, Huuguet F, Laethem JL, et al. Effect of chemoradiotherapy vs chemotherapy on survival in patients with locally advanced pancreatic cancer controlled after 4 months of gemcitabine with or without erlotinib: The LAP07 randomized clinical trial. JAMA. 2016;**315**(17):1844-1853

[30] Ferrone CR, Marchegiani G, Hong TS, et al. Radiological and surgical implications of neoadjuvant treatment with FOLFIRINOX for locally advanced and borderline resectable pancreatic cancer. Annals of Surgery. 2015;**261**(1): 12-17

[31] Blazer M, Wu C, Goldberg RM, et al. Neoadjuvant mFOLFIRINOX for locally advanced unresectable (LAPC) and borderline resectable (BRPC) adenocarcinoma of the pancreas. Annals of Surgical Oncology. 2015;**22**(40): 1153-1159

[32] Amer AM, Zais M, Chaudhury B, et al. Imaging-based biomarkers: Changes in the tumor interface of pancreatic ductal adenocarcinoma on computed tomography scans indicate response to cytotoxic therapy. Cancer. 2018;**124**(8):1701-1709

[33] He J, Blair AB, Groot VP, et al. Is a pathological complete response following neoadjuvant chemoradiation associated with prolonged survival in patients with pancreatic cancer? Annals of Surgery. 2018;**268**(1):1-8

[34] Martin RC. Use of irreversible electroporation in unresectable pancreatic cancer. Hepatobiliary Surgery and Nutrition. 2015;**4**(3): 211-215

[35] Cleary J. Niraparib in patients with pancreatic cancer. ClinicalTrials.gov Identifier: NCT03601923. 2018. Retrieved from: https://clinicaltrials.gov/ct2/show/NCT03601923

[36] Hong TS. Losartan and nivolumab in combination with FOLFIRINOX and SBRT in localized pancreatic cancer. ClinicalTrials.gov Identifier: NCT03563248. 2018. Retrieved from: https://clinicaltrials.gov/ct2/show/NCT03563248

[37] Katz MHG, Herman JM, Ahmad SA, et al. Alliance for clinical trials in oncology (ALLIANCE) trial A021501: preoperative extended chemotherapy vs. chemotherapy plus hypofractionated radiation therapy for borderline resectable adenocarcinoma of the head of the pancreas. BMC Cancer. 2017; **17**(1):505

[38] Chang DT. Phase III FOLFIRINOX (mFFX) +/– SBRT in locally advanced pancreatic cancer. ClinicalTrials.gov Identifier: NCT01926197. 2013. Retrieved from: https://clinicaltrials.gov/ct2/show/NCT01926197

[39] Hubbard JH, Grothey A. Napabucasin: An update on the first-in-class cancer stemness inhibitor. Drugs. 2017;**77**(10):1091-1103

Chapter 4

Colon Cancer

Mehmet Ali Koc, Suleyman Utku Celik and Cihangir Akyol

Abstract

Colorectal cancers (CRCs) are commonly diagnosed malignancy in both men and women. Although it is a common disease, mortality rates decrease with widespread use of screening methods and novel developments in surgery. Physical examination, abdomen and pelvic computerized tomography, and chest imaging are necessary for preoperative staging and surgical planning of a newly diagnosed colon cancer. CRCs usually develop from adenomatous polyps. Although curative treatment of localized colon cancer is surgery, endoscopic polypectomy is sufficient when severe dysplasia or carcinoma in situ is detected on a polyp surface. Total mesorectal excision and neoadjuvant chemoradiotherapy in rectum cancers resulted in significant reductions in morbidity, mortality, and recurrence rates. Recently, complete mesocolic excision and central vascular ligation method has been described in the surgical treatment of colon cancer to achieve similar results. Unfortunately, metastatic colon cancer rate at presentation is approximately 20%. Surgery is a potentially curative option in selected patients with liver and lung metastasis. Pathologic stage of the tumor at presentation is the most important prognostic factor after resection. Therefore, early diagnosis of colon cancer by screening methods and new surgical techniques will lead to better results in survival rates.

Keywords: colon cancer, central vascular ligation, complete mesocolic excision, prevention, treatment

1. Introduction

Colorectal cancer (CRC) is the second most common cancer in women and third in men with an estimation of approximately 1.4 million new cases globally [1]. Men are more affected than women in most of the world with a higher incidence in North America and Europe and, lower incidence in South-Central Asia and Africa [1]. Although it is a common disease, mortality rates decrease with novel developments in surgery and widespread use of screening methods such as colonoscopy, computed tomography colonoscopy, fecal occult blood test. In the United States, decrease in CRC mortality rates has been shown in the Survey of Epidemiology and End Results (SEER) program [2]. Due to comprehensive researches about the biological and molecular characteristics of CRC, cancer pathogenesis has been well elucidated. Since CRC develops after a long process under the influence of both genetic and environmental factors, early diagnosis is possible and as a result there are better treatment outcomes and prognosis [1–3].

Colorectal cancer incidence rises steadily after the age of 50 years and most of the cases are diagnosed in 6th and 7th decades. The incidence under age 40 years is only 5% [3]. Although it is recommended to initiate screening studies at 50 years age, suspicious symptoms like rectal bleeding, unexplained anemia, change in bowel habits, and weight loss should be investigated regardless of the individual's age. Approximately 80% of CRCs are sporadic, 15% are non-syndromic familial, and 5% are syndromic familial cancers [3–5].

CRC is more common in developed societies that consume high-calorie diets rich in animal fat, red meat, processed meat, sweets, refined grains, and alcohol. However a diet rich in fiber, vegetables, fruits, fish, dairy products, and olive oil is beneficial to prevent CRC [4, 5]. The consumption of vegetable fibers shortens the period of contact of the carcinogenic substances with the colon mucosa and at the same time increases the fecal volume and leads to the dilution of the harmful substances so that the adverse effect on the mucosa is reduced. The fat-rich diet stimulates bile acid and cholesterol synthesis in the liver, the amount of these sterols in the colon increases. Due to colon bacteria, production of secondary bile acids and other toxic metabolites are increased and causes negative effects on the colon mucosa [3, 6]. The intake of A, C, E vitamins, calcium, selenium, and carotenoids is thought to reduce the risk of developing CRC [5, 6]. The risk of developing CRC in obese and sedentary individuals also increases like other cancers [7]. Furthermore, chronic alcohol consumption and smoking have been reported to increase the risk of colon adenomas.

The risk of developing CRC in individuals with long-standing inflammatory bowel disease is significantly increased [8]. It is thought that chronic inflammation of the mucosa is a predisposing factor for CRC. Extent and the duration of the colitis is closely related with the development of CRC. While the cumulative risk of CRC in ulcerative colitis patients with pancolitis or left-sided disease is 1.6% at 10 years, it increases approximately 5 times at 20 years (8.3%), and 11 times at 30 years (18.4%) [9]. A similar risk for CRC is also associated with Crohn's disease. Screening colonoscopy for CRC has been recommended annually for patients with inflammatory bowel disease, 8–10 years after the first symptoms of the disease [10].

2. Pathogenesis

Most CRCs usually develop from adenomatous polyps that become dysplastic (adenoma-carcinoma sequence) (**Figures 1** and **2**). The epithelium of small bowel is constantly renewed. During this renewal process, progressive deterioration leads primarily to adenomatous polyps and later to dysplasia and invasive cancer. Hypothesis that CRC are a result of adenoma-carcinoma sequence are supported by findings such as frequent early carcinoma detection in large adenomatous polyps, detection of adenomas in patients 10 years before cancer in both sporadic and familial cases, and reduction of CRC incidence by removal of polyps in controlled trials [11].

CRCs occur by accumulation of epigenetic and genetic changes over time [12]. These changes transform normal glandular epithelium into adenocarcinoma. In hereditary forms of CRC, individuals are born with mutant genes. That means the mutant gene is present in one allele in the zygote from the beginning (germ-line mutation) but a second hit needed. Hereditary non-polyposis colorectal cancer (HNPCC) and familial adenomatous polyposis (FAP) are the best known types of hereditary CRC. Sometimes mutations develop after birth due to environmental factors (somatic mutation) and sporadic cancers occur [10–13].

Tumor suppressor gene mutations may remove an inhibitory signal while oncogenic mutations may cause overexpression of a gene or pathway [11]. These changes

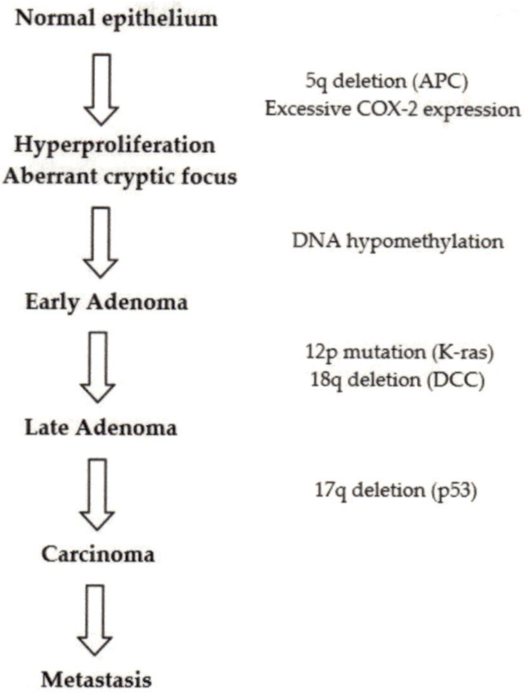

Figure 1.
Adenoma—carcinoma sequence.

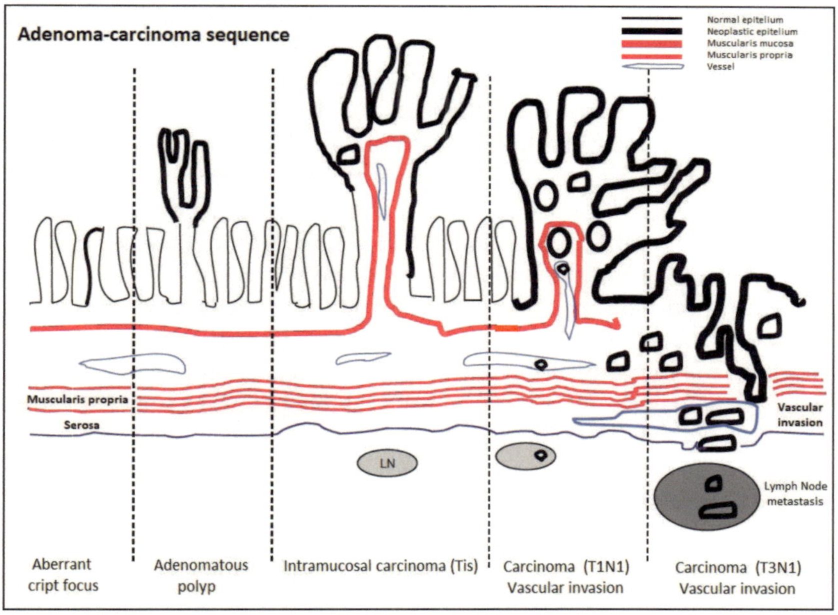

Figure 2.
Adenoma—carcinoma sequence (figure taken from with permission of Prof. Kuzu, Turkish Society of Colon and Rectal Surgery; Colon and Rectum Cancers.Eds, Baykan A, Zorluoglu A, Gecim E, Terzi C. 2010).

that cause CRC, which is a different heterogenous disease in each person, affect the phenotype of the disease, prognosis and response to treatment. Chromosomal instability, microsatellite instability, and the methylator phenotype are the three major molecular pathways that involved in CRC development.

Each pathway has unique characteristics, and multiple pathways may play a role in the development of CRC [12, 13].

2.1 Chromosomal instability

Chromosomes are unstable in chromosomal instability (CIN), because of a change in the chromosome structure or copy number (Loss of heterozygosity-LOH). CIN is the most common occurrence in CRC [13]. Approximately 80% of CRC patients have CIN. Vogelstein and Fearon described the classical adenoma-carcinoma sequence and their study supported that LOH was responsible for the sequence [14]. The main genes which play role in the carcinogenesis are the adenomatous polyposis coli (APC), K-ras, deleted in colon cancer (DCC), and P53 (**Figure 1**).

The APC is a tumor suppressor gene, therefore, mutation in both alleles are necessary for the initiation of the sequence. Mutated APC causes decreased production or lack of APC protein. Thus, translocation into the nucleus due to intracellular accumulation of β-caterin, which is controlled by the APC protein to regulate the WNT signaling pathway, causes alterations in cell signaling, proliferation, and adhesion [15]. The APC gene is first described in patients with FAP. However, it was then reported that majority of the sporadic CRC has the APC gene mutation and APC mutation is present in adenomas smaller than 0.5 cm [16].

K-ras is a cellular variant of RAS oncogenes and the most frequently mutated RAS proto-oncogene in CRC. Since K-ras is a proto-oncogene, mutation of only one allele is enough. K-ras gene encodes a G-protein (Guanine nucleotide binding protein) that is active when GTP bond state and inactive (GDP-bond state) after hydrolyzed by GTPase. This protein is involved in mitogen-activated protein kinase (MAPK) pathway which promotes cell growth and proliferation. RAS mutation results in an active GTP-bond protein, which is unable to switch off by GTPase, and leads to uncontrolled cell division. About 43% of non-hypermutated (Microsatellite stabile-MSS) CRC, which are nearly 80% of CRC, has RAS mutations [17].

DCC and SMAD4 mutations have been found in CRCs [18, 19]. Both are tumor suppressor genes. DCC gene product is thought to be involved in cell differentiation and adhesion in CRC [20]. *DCC* and SMAD4 (formerly PC4-deleted in pancreatic cancer) were both identified at 18q. SMAD4 mutations is thought to perturb TGF-beta signaling pathway which has an inhibitory influence on normal cell growth [19, 20].

TP53 gene on chromosome 17p encode P53 protein which arrests the cell cycle and facilitates DNA repair [21]. In all human cancers most of the mutations occur in TP53 gene. TP53 mutation occurs in about 75% of CRCs [14]. However it is not frequent in adenomas, therefore, it is considered to be a late event in CRC tumorigenesis and related with invasiveness [22, 23].

2.2 Microsatellite instability (MSI)

Microsatellites are non-coding DNA segments containing 1 to 4 repetitive nucleotide sequences. In normal individuals microsatellites are completely identical in all cells. But the failure of the DNA mismatch repair genes to function properly causes a change in the length of the microsatellite sites that are already prone to error during copying. This is called microsatellite instability. There are also short repetitive segments in various tumor suppressor genes (TSG), and accumulation of the mutations in TSGs due to the inactivity of MMR genes (most commonly MLH1 or MSH2) lead to the development of adenoma and subsequent carcinoma [21–23].

It is possible to detect microsatellite instability with current diagnostic procedures, as long as many cells carry the same abnormality, which means that the cells belong to the clonal process. Clonal proliferation is a characteristic feature of the neoplastic process. And It should be understood that MSI is an indicator of a clonal neoplastic process [24].

Cancers arising through MSI pathway are approximately 15% of all CRC and tend to be hypermutated, therefore, are also termed the mutator phenotype [17]. However, prognosis is better than cancers arising through CIN pathway.

2.3 CpG island methylator phenotype (CIMP)

Another common pathway in CRC is epigenetic instability. Epigenetic alterations such as hypermethylation of DNA promoter regions can silence gene transcription and contributes to diseases like cancer. Methylation of cytosine is normally an essential process and controls multiple processes [25]. There are cytosine-guanine (CpG) dinucleotide enriched areas in promoter regions. These CpG enriched regions of genes are called CpG islands and normally maintained in an unmethylated state. Several tumor suppressor genes contain CpG repetitive sequences in the promoter region. Aberrant methylation of these CpG islands silences gene transcription and contributes to cancer process [25, 26]. This phenomenon is called CpG island methylator phenotype (CIMP). Especially methylation of the MMR gene, hMLH1 causes approximately 80% of MSI CRCs [27]. Almost all MSI-high (MSI–H), CIMP+ cancers without K-ras mutations have BRAF mutations. However, Lynch-related CRCs only have K-ras mutations [28, 29].

3. Hereditary colorectal cancers

3.1 Hereditary non-polyposis colorectal cancer (HNPCC)

HNPCC is the most common hereditary colorectal cancer. HNPCC is also termed Lynch syndrome. In Lynch syndrome, CRC and endometrial cancer risk are significantly increased as well as several other malignancies. It accounts for 3% of all colorectal cancers [30]. Lynch is an autosomal dominant disease. Mutations in DNA repair genes (mismatch repair-MMR) are detected in affected individuals. In Lynch syndrome there is a germline mutation. Since this mutation is only in one allele, a second hit is necessary (mutation, loss of heterozygosity, or epigenetic silencing). Colorectal cancer develops in 80% of patients around 40 years of age. The most frequently mutated MMR genes in HNPCC were MLH 1 (37%), MSH 2 (41%), MSH 6, and PMS 2. CRCs developed in Lynch syndrome are MSI-H tumors [30].

In patients with Lynch syndrome, the risk of synchronous and metachronous tumors is increased, and approximately 7% of patients have a second tumor at the time of diagnosis [31]. Metachronous tumors develop within 10 years in 16% of individuals who had previously undergone colon resection due to Lynch syndrome and within 30 years this rate reaches to 62% [32].

Lynch-associated CRCs also evolve from adenomas like most CRCs. However the adenomas are more often proximally located, and more likely to be larger and flatter. And as compared with sporadic adenomas, high-grade dysplasia and/or villous histology are more often detected. It is also known that the adenoma-carcinoma sequence progresses more rapidly in Lynch syndrome. Fortunately, the overall 10-year survival from CRC is 91% [33].

Tumors in HNPCC are more often found in the proximal colon than sporadic cancers. Unlike sporadic cancers, tumor in Lynch is poor differentiated and there is peritumoral lymphocytic infiltration, and Crohn's-like reaction [34]. However, the prognosis is still better than sporadic colorectal cancer. The following three theories stand out for this reason: earlier diagnosis in HNPCC tumors, the genomic instability in HNPCC tumors leads to the continual increase of mutations and the loss of critical functions and metastatic ability of the tumor cell due to this mutation burden, and Crohn's-like lymphocytic infiltration around the tumor enhances host immunity by expressing IL-4, TNF-a [33, 34].

Two different forms of HNPCC have been described. Lynch Syndrome I is characterized with proximal colon tumor, young age, no extracolonic involvement. Generally same colonic segment is involved in other relatives. In Lynch Syndrome II, in addition to Lynch I, stomach, small intestine, pancreas, ovary, endometrium and urinary tract cancers may develop. The most important tool in diagnosing Lynch syndrome is family history of CRC or other cancers related with Lynch. Several family history-based criteria (Revised Bethesda Guidelines and Amsterdam II Criteria) have been used to determine the people at risk for HNPCC (**Table 1**) [34].

MSI is a characteristic of tumors in HNPCC and caused by a loss of DNA MMR. An MSI screening test is required for patients with a positive Bethesda criteria. Polymerase chain reaction is used to test for MSI by copying a panel of DNA sequences that contains nucleotide repeats [33–35]. Family members who meet the Amsterdam II criteria or revised Bethesda guidelines, or those with a diagnosis of endometrium cancer prior to the age of 50 years, or individuals with a MMR gene mutation in the first degree relatives are at risk for Lynch syndrome.

In Lynch syndrome, synchronous or metachronous cancer and polyp development are common. It is important to be cautious in this regard. Colonoscopy should be done every one or two years starting from the age of 20–25 [36, 37]. Gynecological examination and endometrial aspiration biopsy for endometrium cancer, and transvaginal ultrasonography for ovarian cancer should be done once a

Amsterdam II Criteria and Revised Bethesda Guidelines

Amsterdam II Criteria [35]

All criteria must be met:

- Three or more individuals with colorectal cancers or HNPCC-related cancers, and one of them being a first-degree relative of the other two,
- Two or more successive generations are affected,
- At least one relative has colorectal or HNPCC-related cancer diagnosed before the age of 50 years.

Revised Bethesda Guidelines [34]

One or more of the following criteria must be met:

- Colorectal cancer diagnosed before the age of 50 years,
- Synchronous or metachronous colorectal cancer or other HNPCC-related tumors*, regardless of age,
- Colorectal cancer with MSI-high histology** diagnosed before the age of 60 years
- Colorectal cancer diagnosed in one or more first degree relatives with HNPCC-related tumor, and one of them being diagnosed before the age of 50 years,
- Colorectal cancer in 2 or more first- or second-degree relatives with HNPCC-associated tumors, regardless of age.

HNPCC: hereditary nonpolyposis colorectal cancer; MSI: microsatellite instability.
**HNPCC-related tumors include colorectal, endometrial, stomach, ovarian, pancreas, ureter and renal pelvis, biliary tract, and brain (usually glioblastoma as seen in Turcot syndrome) tumors, sebaceous gland adenomas and keratoacanthomas in Muir-Torre syndrome, and carcinoma of the small bowel.*
***Presence of tumor-infiltrating lymphocytes, Crohn's-like lymphocytic reaction, mucinous/signet-ring cell differentiation, or medullary growth pattern.*

Table 1.
Amsterdam II Criteria and Revised Bethesda Guidelines.

year starting from the age of 30–35, or 3–5 years prior to the age of a relative diagnosed with HNPCC [37]. Upper gastrointestinal endoscopy should be done once every 2 years starting from the age of 30–35, with gastric biopsy and treatment for *Helicobacter pylori* infection when found on biopsy. Renal ultrasound, urine analysis and cytology should be done every year starting from the age of 30–35 [36, 37].

3.1.1 Treatment

Prophylactic colectomy is not considered in patients without CRC. Tumor is usually located in the proximal colon. Total abdominal colectomy—ileorectal anastomosis is recommended in patients with Lynch syndrome. Considering the quality of life in elderly patients, or in patients who are not eligible for total colectomy a segmental colectomy may be recommended according to the location of the tumor [36]. However patients who undergo segmental colectomy are at increased risk for subsequent CRC as compared to patients with total abdominal colectomy—ileorectal anastomosis [38, 39]. Prophylactic hysterectomy and oophorectomy should be recommended at the time of colorectal surgery. However, it may be recommended for women who aged 35 years or older after family planning [39].

3.2 Familial adenomatous polyposis (FAP)

It accounts for 1% of all colorectal cancers and is an autosomal dominant disease. FAP is characterized by the presence of hundreds of adenomas in the colon (**Figure 3**). It is a broad spectrum disease with extraintestinal manifestations. It usually occurs after puberty and is diagnosed at a mean age of 29 years. Colorectal cancer develops at an average age of 39 years. Colorectal cancer is unavoidable in patients who do not undergo surgery. FAP is 80% familial, and 20% sporadic [40].

Mutation in the APC (adenomatous polyposis coli) gene, which is located at the q21 locus of chromosome 5, is responsible for FAP (5q deletion) [40, 41]. Mutations in codons close to the 3'and 5' ends of the APC gene lead to attenuated FAP (AFAP), while mutations in the middle, between codons 169 to 1393, result in FAP. Generally, there is less than 100 polyps in AFAP. Unlike FAP, life-long risk for CRC development in AFAP is approximately 70%, and polyps and CRCs develop later in life than FAP. In AFAP, tumors mostly do not develop in the rectum and are characterized by a more proximal distribution in the colon. If germline mutation is absent in these patients, MMR gene mutation should be considered for HNPCC elimination [41]. In

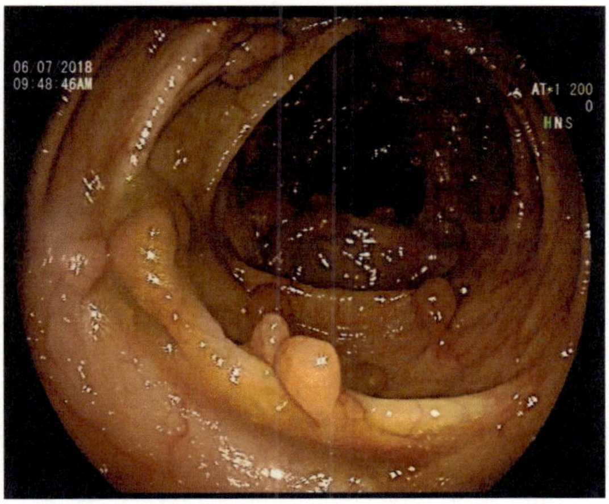

Figure 3.
Colonoscopic familial adenomatous polyposis (FAP).

FAP, one inherited mutant allele is not enough to cause carcinoma. Carcinoma develops when the second allele of APC and other necessary gene mutations occur [42].

Extraintestinal manifestations of FAP include gastric, duodenal, and periampullary polyps, and less common manifestations such as epidermoid cysts, desmoid tumors, osteomas, and brain tumors. Gastric and duodenal polyps occur in about half of affected individuals. Most of the gastric polyps are hyperplasia of the fundus glands, rather than adenomatous polyps and their malignancy potential is limited [43]. However duodenal polyps are adenomatous. They are present in approximately 90% of FAP patients and should be considered premalignant [44, 45]. Periampullary tumor risk is higher in FAP patients. In patients who undergo total colectomy, the most important cause of cancer-related death is duodenal adenocancer. Adenomatous polyps and cancer are rarely found in the jejunum and ileum of FAP patients. Other rare extraintestinal malignancies in FAP patients are extrahepatic bile duct, gallbladder, pancreas, adrenal, thyroid, and liver cancers [45].

The likelihood of a desmoid tumor is increased especially in mutations in the 3‘ end of the APC gene [46]. Most of the desmoid tumors occur within the first 5 years in patients who have undergone abdominal surgery, presumably as an inflammatory response [47, 48]. In addition to abdominal surgery and APC mutation, pregnancy, female sex, and family history are other risk factors for desmoid tumors [49, 50]. Although desmoid tumors are slow growing, non-metastatic mesenchymal tumors, they may cause complications such as pain, bowel, and ureter obstruction by compressing and encasing adjacent structures [50].

An interesting marker for FAP is congenital hypertrophy of the retinal pigment epithelium (CHRPE), which can be determined by ophthalmoscopy in about 75% of patients [51]. Fundus examination with ophthalmoscopy reveals oval, pigmented lesions with regular borders in the retina. Lesions may be bilateral and multiple. CHRPE can be used as a clinical diagnostic tool in the screening of FAP and Gardner syndrome [51].

FAP has two subtypes with their own extracolonic manifestations. Gardner's syndrome is a variant of FAP and characterized by desmoid tumors, colonic polyps, osteoma, soft tissue sarcomas, and CHRPE [52]. Also, although very rare, an adenomatous polyposis coli may be associated with malignant tumors of the central nervous system (especially medulloblastoma and/or glioma), known as Turcot syndrome [53]. Turcot is the true variant form of FAP and has a familial character. Colonoscopy and brain scanning tests should also be performed on family members. APC mutations are also responsible for both syndromes.

Screening for FAP should be performed in individuals with an APC mutation and in individuals who are first-degree relatives of those with FAP, or who have >10 cumulative colorectal adenomas, or colorectal adenomas in combination with extracolonic features such as duodenal adenomas, desmoid tumors, osteomas, etc. [53, 54].

Screening for CRC should begin during puberty and flexible sigmoidoscopy, or genetic testing for APC mutations should be performed every 6 months or year. When positive genotype is detected by genetic screening, or adenomatous polyps are detected by sigmoidoscopy, full colonoscopy should be performed to evaluate the spread of the disease. Several polyps should also be sampled to confirm histology. First-degree relatives of FAP patients, who do not have a genetic diagnosis, may be removed from aggressive follow-up and included in standard general population screening programs if there is no polyp detected until 40 years of age on screening [54]. Screening of the upper gastrointestinal tract should be performed at the time of diagnosis, or before 25 years of age. In later periods, it should be done while the colon is being evaluated. Thyroid cancer is rarely seen in patients with FAP. Studies have shown that thyroid cancer reaches up to 2.6% and thyroid nodules up to 51.7%. Therefore, it is recommended to screen thyroid gland by ultrasonography once a year [55, 56].

3.2.1 Genetic testing

Identification of the APC mutation and its type in a patient diagnosed with FAP facilitates screening of other family members as well as recognition of possible phenotypic lesions that may result from different APC mutations. Commonly accepted indications for genetic testing include FAP cases, FAP in first degree relatives, APC mutation in first degree relatives, at least 10 cumulative colorectal adenomas, extracolonic involvement of FAP and multiple adenomas with colorectal cancer family history but without a FAP trait in the family [36].

3.2.2 Treatment

3.2.2.1 Medical treatment and chemoprevention

In cases with FAP non-steroid anti-inflammatory drugs (NSAIDs) are thought to achieve regression in number and size of polyps [57, 58]. The most commonly used agents for this purpose are sulindac and celecoxib. The role of chemopreventive agents in FAP patients is controversial, because the effects of these agents on cancer prevention are unclear.

3.2.2.2 Surgical treatment

Prophylactic colectomy should be performed in all cases with FAP. The timing of surgery is planned according to the number of polyps, number of adenomas, presence of dysplasia, size of polyps, symptoms and characteristics of the patient. In cases with mild to moderate polyposis and no other risk factors (low risk of cancer), surgery can be done at mid-puberty. However patients should continue to undergo annual CRC surveillance with colonoscopy while awaiting colectomy. Surgery should be performed in patients with severe polyposis, dysplasia, and polyp greater than 5 mm and in symptomatic cases without any time loss after diagnosis [58].

Surgical treatment options include subtotal colectomy with ileorectal anastomosis (IRA), total proctocolectomy with ileal pouch-anal anastomosis (IPAA), or total proctocolectomy and permanent ileostomy. Total proctocolectomy and permanent ileostomy is preferred in cases of rectal tumor that involved the sphincter complex, and in cases which IPAA is not technically feasible. Functional outcomes (quality of life) and the risk of developing rectal cancer, which is the result of leaving the rectum in place, are important in the selection of anorectal anastomosis or IPAA. Patients with a few rectal polyps which can be controlled endoscopically are ideal for IRA. Chemoprevention is recommended for these patients in the postoperative period. Since colon cancer mostly develops in proximal colon in AFAP patients, total abdominal colectomy and IRA is ideal for this group [58–60].

Risks of developing rectal cancer in the 10th and 25th years in patients undergoing IRA are 4–8% and 26–30% respectively [59, 60]. It is known that adenoma or cancer may develop in patients with IPAA, even in those with end ileostomy [61]. Therefore, the remaining rectum or pouch should be examined endoscopically at 6 months or 1 year intervals after whichever method is preferred (IPAA, IRA). IRA should be avoided in cases with family history of desmoid tumor, and IPAA should be preferred. Because in the case of a cancer or polyposis that may develop later in the rectum, revision of IRA to IPAA would be technically very difficult due to mesenteric desmoids that may develop [54].

3.3 MutYH-associated polyposis (MAP)

The number of polyps may range from 0 to 1000, but it is known that MAP usually contains less adenomatous polyps than FAP. MAP is an autosomal recessive disease. There is a biallelic mutation of the MutYH (MYH) gene on chromosome 1 [62]. MAP usually occurs in fifth or sixth decade with a polyp number of 10–100 [62, 63]. There are insufficient data on extraintestinal manifestations. However, gastric and duodenal polyps may be found in individuals with MAP. Unlike FAP, there is no association with desmoids, osteomas, and CHRPE in MAP [63].

MAP should be suspected in individuals with 10 or more cumulative adenomas as in other adenomatous polyposis syndromes. Germline MYH testing is recommended to those who have a family history of colorectal cancer or polyposis in recessive pattern, or who have a clinical FAP or AFAP phenotype but a negative APC mutation test result. In patients with biallelic MUTYH mutations, the cumulative lifetime risk of developing colorectal cancer is 75% in men and 72% in women by age 70 [64]. Most of the patients with MAP are diagnosed when they have cancer, but it is recommended to perform a colonoscopy every one to two years to individuals with known biallelic mutations, starting at 25–30 years of age [36].

CRC, adenomatous polyp with high-grade dysplasia that cannot be removed endoscopically, and a great number of polyps that cannot be controlled endoscopically are indications for surgery. It is recommended to remove the newly developed polyps by performing at least annual colonoscopy in patients not eligible for surgery. Surgical options include subtotal colectomy with IRA, total abdominal colectomy, or proctocolectomy with IPAA [63, 64].

4. Clinical findings of colon cancer

Patients frequently present with changes in bowel habits, rectal bleeding, anemia, and abdominal pain accompanying these findings. Patients may also suffer from weight loss, fatigue, nausea, vomiting, obstruction and perforation [65–69]. Clinical findings vary according to the tumor location. Abdominal pain, which can be seen in all localizations, is the most common clinical manifestation. The most common symptoms in right colon tumors are blunt, permanent lower quadrant pain and anemia of iron deficiency due to occult hemorrhage, fatigue, and anorexia and weight loss. Sometimes, a mass can be palpated in the lower right quadrant [24, 68, 69].

In the left colon, the diameter is smaller (especially sigmoid colon) and the content is solid. In addition, left colon cancers are scirrhous and annular. Therefore, obstructive symptoms are common. Obstruction may lead to perforation and peritonitis. According to Laplace's law, the most likely location of perforation as a result of obstruction of the sigmoid colon is the cecum of which the diameter is largest. A change in bowel habits and a progressive decrease in stool diameter may be the first symptoms. While rectal bleeding may be a finding as occult blood in feces on the right side, it may occur as hematochezia on the left side. In the presence of iron deficiency anemia in an adult male or postmenopausal woman, the diagnosis of colon cancer should be absolutely ruled out [67–70].

Patients may also present with metastatic disease. At the time of presentation, metastatic disease is detected in approximately 20 percent of patients in the United States [70]. Advanced, or often metastatic disease should be suspected in case of the presence of abdominal distention, ascites, early satiety, right upper quadrant pain, periumbilical nodules, or supraclavicular lymphadenopathy.

Colon cancer can spread in 4 different ways; directly through the neighborhood, lymphatic route, hematogen route, and through the peritoneal cavity by

DOI: http://dx.doi.org/10.5772/intechopen.81597

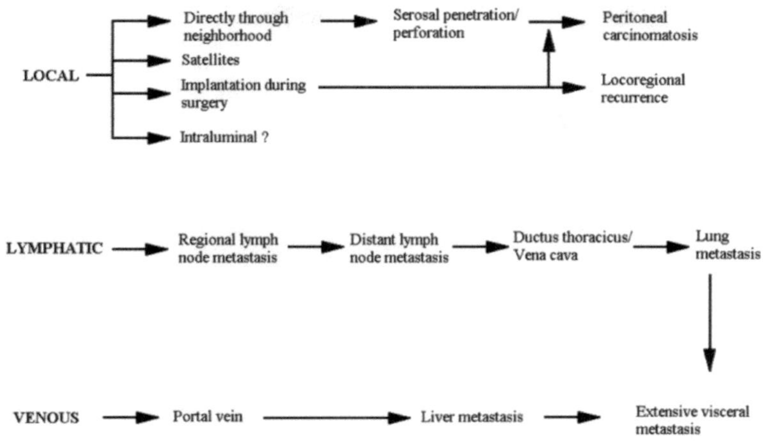

Figure 4.
Colon cancer dissemination.

gravity (seeding) (**Figure 4**). It should be remembered that tumor may also spread by implantation due to manipulation at the time of surgery. The most common metastasis is in the regional lymph nodes. The most important factor determining lymph node involvement is the T category. While lymph node metastasis is 5–20% in T1–T2 tumors, in T3–T4 tumors lymph node involvement increases to more than 50%. Tumor differentiation, presence of lymphovascular invasion and tumor size are other factors. Hematogenous spread occurs with portal system and the most common site for metastasis is the liver. The other common sites for metastasis after liver is the lung and bones. Seeding is caused by the placement of free tumor cells in the omentum, periton (peritoneal carcinomatosis), rectovesical pouch (Blumer's shelf tumors), and ovary (Krukenberg tumors) [70, 71].

5. Diagnosis and preoperative evaluation in colon cancer

Colon cancer may be suspected from vague but suspicious symptoms and signs, or sometimes, especially asymptomatic CRC, may only be revealed by routine screening. Anamnesis, physical and rectal examination are valuable in diagnosis. If there is a suspicion of CRC in the patient after anamnesis and physical examination, the first diagnostic test should be colonoscopy or flexible sigmoidoscopy. In addition, barium enema and computed tomography colonography (CTC) may be performed, if necessary.

The most accurate and preferred diagnostic test for colon cancer is colonoscopy since it can be used for detecting and sampling of lesions along the large bowel, examination of lesions by direct observation, treatment in appropriate patients, and detection of synchronous tumors. Synchronous CRCs occur in 4–5% of patients [71, 72]. In some individuals, a minority of neoplastic lesions are nonpolypoid and flat, and may be more challenging to detect by colonoscopy. However colonoscopy is still more sensitive in this situation than barium enema or CTC [72].

Flexible rectosigmoidoscopy can be used for diagnostic purposes as well. It is mostly recommended for screening of CRC every 5 years, starting at the age of 50 with annual fecal occult blood test. In recent years there is an increase in right-sided or proximal colon cancers. Because of this and the likelihood of synchronous CRCs, it should be considered that flexible sigmoidoscopy may be an inadequate test for diagnosis of a patient suspected of having a CRC [72, 73].

Computerized tomography is the most frequently used test for staging purposes. Positron emission tomography has no place in routine staging and screening. However, in suspicious cases, tumor and fibrous tissue are well separated. Abdominal ultrasonography has no place in the diagnosis of colon cancer [71].

Routine laboratory tests including complete blood count, liver function tests, etc. have no role in diagnosis. However In the presence of iron deficiency anemia in an adult male or postmenopausal woman, colon cancer should be ruled out. Although liver function tests has no role in diagnosis of liver metastasis, the increase in liver enzymes in patients with colon cancer should be taken into consideration to scan for metastasis [71, 72].

It is known that some tumor markers, especially CEA (carcinoembryonic antigen), are associated with CRC. Nevertheless, tumor markers such as CEA and CA 19-9 appears to have a low diagnostic yield to diagnose primary CRC, since these markers have low sensitivity for early-stage disease and may also increase in some benign diseases. However, both markers have prognostic significance. High CEA suggests the presence of metastasis. In addition, after appropriate treatment increase in CEA level in follow-up should be assessed in favor of recurrence or metastasis [73].

6. Staging

The local features (size, invasion, lymph node involvement) of the tumor are important in determining the resection margin. Therefore, preoperative clinical staging should be done properly. Physical examination and radiological tests are used for accurate clinical staging. It should not be forgotten that the accuracy of radiological detection of the stage is 85–90%, even in the best hands. Definitive staging can only be performed by pathological examination [74].

Pathologic staging in colorectal cancers is based on tumor depth, lymph node involvement, and the metastatic status. Dukes and Astler-Coller classifications are no longer used, instead the TNM staging system is preferred [74]. The most recent (8th edition) revision of the TNM staging classification contains few changes compared with the earlier edition (7th edition). T categories have been revised. Tis in the AJCC 8th edition refers only to intramucosal carcinoma, a lesion with involvement of lamina propria with no extension through muscularis mucosae. T4 is defined as tumor exceeds the visceral peritoneum either by continuous invasion or perforation of the tumor. N categories have not changed. Lastly, the M category has been expanded, with the addition of M1c for peritoneal metastases. Therefore, a new stage, IVc, have been added in stage grouping.

Stage of the disease is the most important prognostic parameter that determines the type of surgery and postoperative treatment options in colorectal cancers. Because of the different lymphatic drainage on the intestinal wall, colorectal cancer gains potential to make metastasis only when there is submucosal invasion. For this reason, colorectal carcinoma is diagnosed only in the presence of submucosal invasion [74].

Dukes staging:

Dukes A: Tumor is limited in the bowel wall.

Dukes B: Invasion through the bowel wall but no lymph node involvement.

Dukes C: Lymph node involvement.

Dukes D: Distant metastasis.

Modified Astler-Coller staging:

A: Tumor is limited to mucosa.

B1: Muscularis propria is invaded but not exceeded.

B2: Invades through muscularis propria (subserosal dissemination).

B3: Lesion involves adjacent organs.
C1: B1 + lymph node involvement.
C2: B2 + lymph node involvement.
C3: B3 + lymph node involvement.
D: Distant metastasis.

7. Treatment

Colon cancers mostly develop from polyps. Although curative treatment of localized colon cancer is surgery, endoscopic polypectomy is enough when carcinoma in situ or severe dysplasia presents on the polyp surface. However, surgery should be considered for the treatment of colon cancer especially in patients a polyp that cannot be removed endoscopically, and if there is continuity in resection margin after polypectomy [75].

In the last decade, there have been major changes in colorectal cancer management. Total mesorectal excision and neoadjuvant chemoradiotherapy in rectum cancers resulted in significant reductions in morbidity, mortality, and recurrence rates. Recently, complete mesocolic excision (CME) and central vascular ligation (CVL) (open or laparoscopic) has been described in colon cancer treatment to achieve similar oncological results. In 2007, Hohenberger published the first article on CME with CVL for colon cancer and which was later published in English [75, 76]. The aim of CME with CVL method is to create an intact protective mesocolic fascia and avoid tumor spread within peritoneal cavity by dissection of the visceral fascia from the parietal (retroperitoneal) plane (**Figure 5**). The origin of colonic vessels is well exposed and ligated centrally at their origin using this technique. The specimens are characterized by a greater distance from the tumor to the high vascular tie, higher distance from the closest bowel wall to the high vascular tie, longer length of the colon and larger area of mesentery. Thus, maximum lymphatic tissue harvest is achieved [76, 77]. Increase in the patients who have a high number of lymph nodes, decrease in perioperative morbidity, reduction in local recurrence, and advancement in colon cancer-specific survival rate have been shown in recent studies regarding CME [76, 78–80]. This technique is a matter of controversy in colon surgery. Because longer operating times, autonomic nerve injury, and major vascular damage are disadvantages of routine implementation of CME. Although the technique has improved oncologic data, routine implementation of CME may decrease health-related quality of life (QoL) [76, 80].

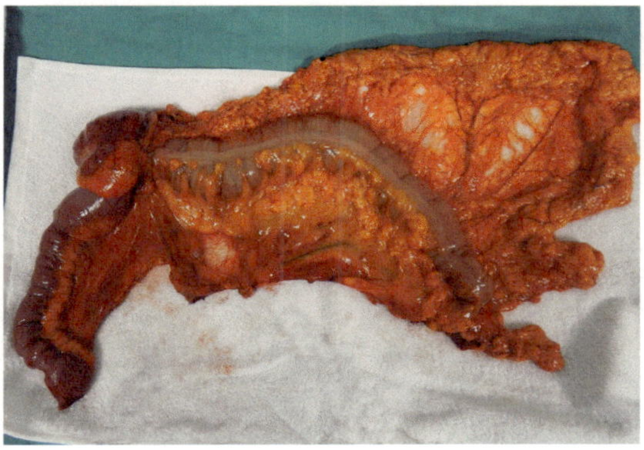

Figure 5.
Complete mesocolic excision and central vascular ligation for the treatment of extended right hemicolectomy specimen.

Surgical resection of the tumor is the main curative treatment option. The colon segment where the tumor is located, the mesentery that contains the lymphatic drainage, and, if there is invasion, adjacent organs should be removed in one piece without deteriorating tumor integrity. If the tumor cannot be removed surgically, palliative surgical procedures such as limited resections, proximal diversion ostomies (colostomy, ileostomy), or bypass surgeries may be applied to relieve symptoms or prevent possible complications [79]. Right hemicolectomy (extended or not), transverse colectomy, left hemicolectomy (extended or not) sigmoid colectomy, and subtotal or total colectomy are preferred for surgical treatments of colon tumors according to involved bowel segment. Surgical intervention may be performed conventional (open) or laparoscopic, provided that it conforms to oncologic principles [80].

7.1 Cecum and ascending colon tumors

Right hemicolectomy is performed as a standard surgical treatment option in the right-sided colon tumors. In this operation, right branch of the middle colic, ileocolic, and right colic vessels are ligated as high as possible. The ascending colon, the hepatic flexure, the first third of the transverse colon, and distal part of the terminal ileum is resected (**Figure 6**). Then, ileocolonic anastomosis is performed between ileum and transverse segment of the colon.

7.2 Hepatic flexure tumors

To remove the entire lymphatic network, CVL of the middle colic, right colic, and ileocolic vessels is performed. This operation is called extended right hemicolectomy (**Figure** 7). When compared to the left hemicolectomy, the amount of transverse colon that is resected increases and only distal 1/3 of the transverse colon is left. An anastomosis should be avoided in areas of unreliable blood supply such as splenic flexure. In this case resection margins should be expanded and splenic

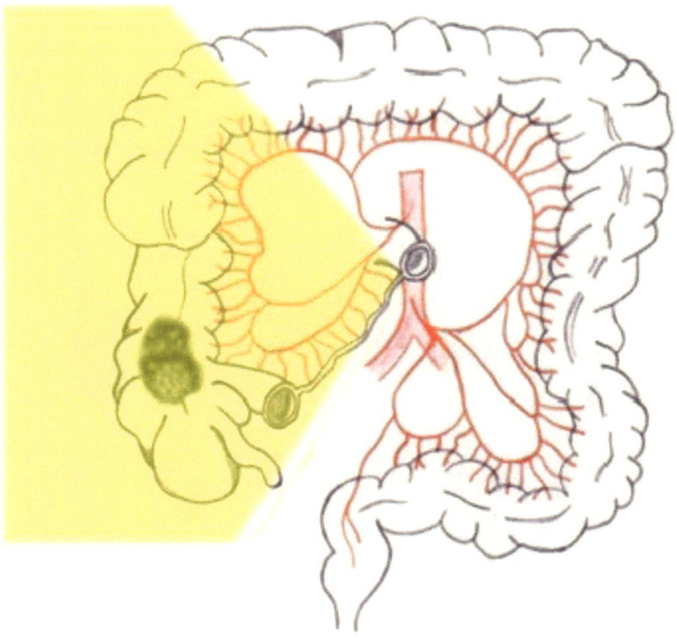

Figure 6.
Resection margins in cecum and ascending colon tumors.

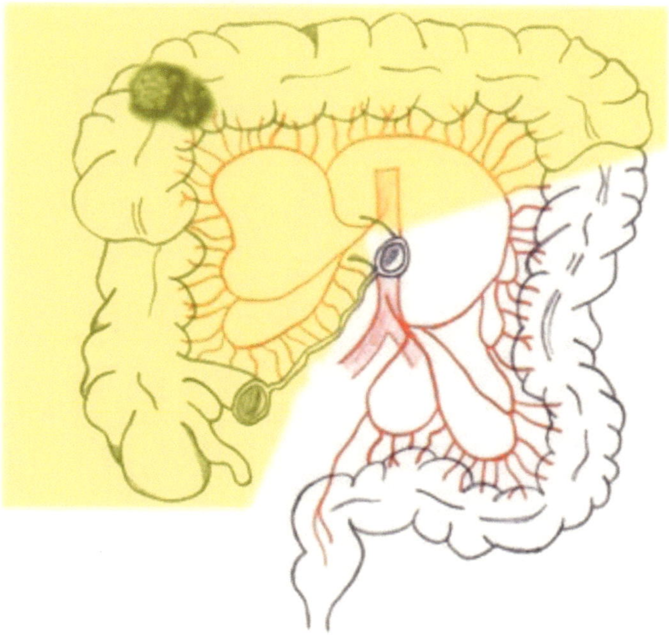

Figure 7.
Resection margins in hepatic flexure tumors.

flexure should be removed as well. Finally, anastomosis is created between the ileum and the proximal end of the remaining colon.

7.3 Transverse colon tumors

The choice of surgery type in transverse colon tumors may be a matter of debate. The arterial supply of the transverse colon is provided by right colic and left colic and middle colic arteries. Ischemia usually does not occur in the anastomosis at the hepatic flexure due to branches from ileocolic and right colic arteries, even if middle colic artery is centrally ligated. However when middle colic artery is ligated, arterial supply of splenic flexure is only provided by left colic artery and there is an ischemia risk in the anastomosis at the splenic flexure. Therefore, transverse colectomy could be performed by CVL of the middle colic and left colic vessels for mid-transverse colon tumors. In this procedure, distal ascending, hepatic flexure, transverse, splenic flexure, and proximal descending colon are resected (**Figure 8**). Moreover, it is recommended surgical resection of the ascending colon and cecum to perform ileosigmoidal anastomosis because it is technically difficult to create an anastomosis between ascending and sigmoid colon. Consequently, it is necessary to consider both the arterial circulation and the lymphatic drainage in the selection of the operation type in transverse colon tumors.

7.4 Splenic flexure tumors

Extended left hemicolectomy is recommended for splenic flexure tumors, as lymphatics may drain to the lymph nodes along the inferior mesenteric artery (IMA) and middle colic artery. The central ligation of the middle colic artery and IMA requires to remove all entire bowel from the proximal transverse colon to the proximal rectum. At the end of the surgical procedure, an anastomosis is performed between proximal transverse colon and proximal segment of the rectum (**Figure 9**).

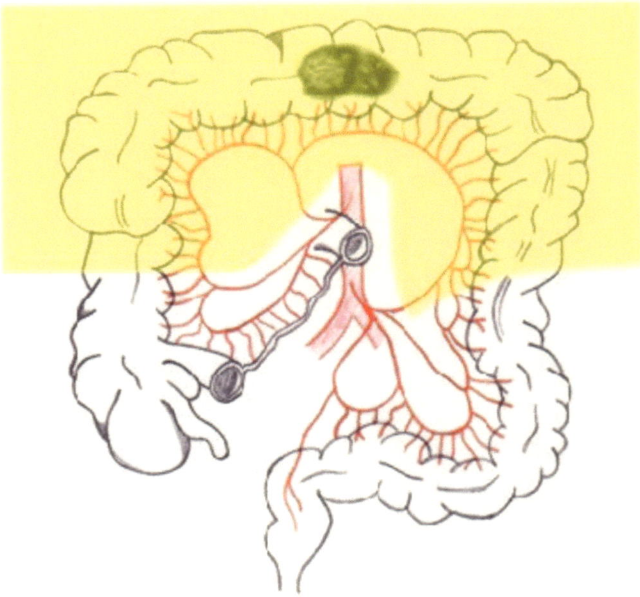

Figure 8.
Resection margins in transverse colon tumors.

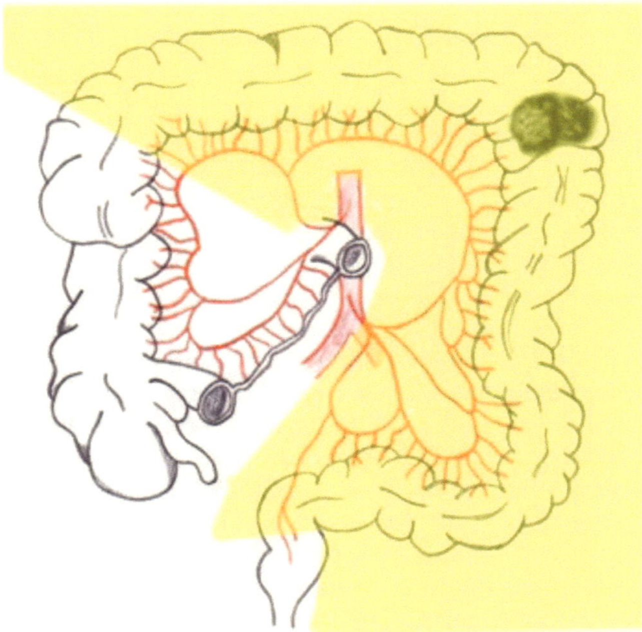

Figure 9.
Resection margins in splenic flexure tumors.

7.5 Descending colon tumors

Left hemicolectomy is recommended in patients with ascending colon tumor. IMA is centrally ligated without preserving the left colic artery. Splenic flexure, descending and sigmoid colons are removed. Then, anastomosis is established between transverse colon and proximal rectum (**Figure 10**).

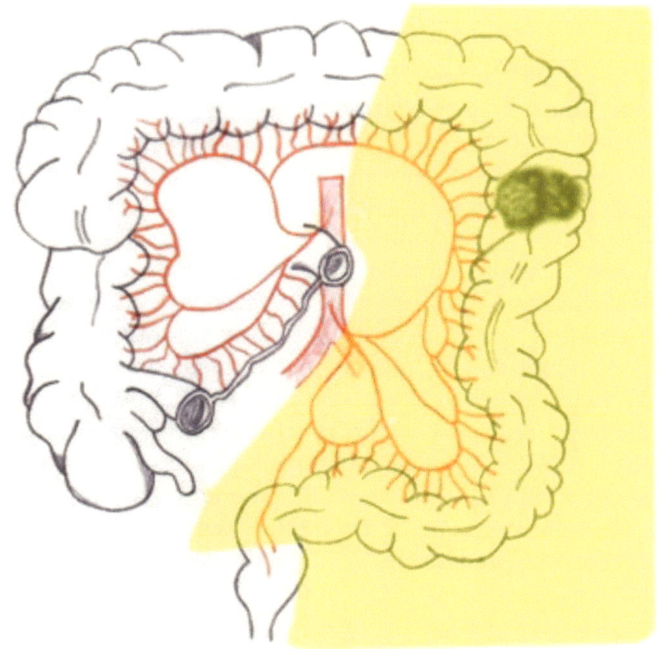

Figure 10.
Resection margins in descending colon tumors.

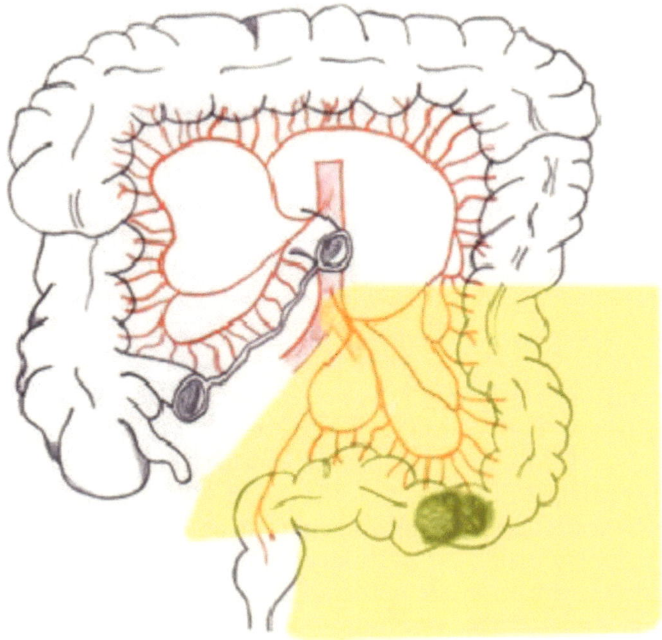

Figure 11.
Resection margins in sigmoid colon tumors.

7.6 Sigmoid colon tumors

The appropriate operation for these tumors is sigmoid colon resection. IMA is centrally ligated while left colic artery is preserved. Sigmoid colon is then removed and colorectal anastomosis is created (**Figure 11**).

8. Prognosis

Pathologic stage at presentation is the strongest prognostic factor. In patients with stage 1 colon tumor, the 5-year survival rate is approximately 90% while it drops to 15% in stage 4 patients [2]. Despite a curative surgery and modern adjuvant treatments, recurrence develops in approximately 40% of stage 2 and 3 patients [81]. Almost all recurrences develop within the first 5 years, and most of them are seen within the first 3 years [82].

Besides pathologic staging, the most important prognostic factors for CRC are histologic grade of differentiation, extramural tumor deposits, lymphovascular and perineural invasion, the preoperative carcinoembryonic antigen (CEA) level, MSI, and *RAS* and *BRAF* mutations. The local extent of disease independently influences survival [83, 84]. However tumor size has no significant impact on prognosis [84, 85]. One of the adverse prognostic factors is residual tumor after resection [86, 87]. There are three types of R designation for residual tumors in non-metastatic patients: R0 resection, complete resection of the tumor with histologically negative margins, R1 resection, incomplete tumor resection with positive microscopic margin involvement, R2 resection, and incomplete resection with macroscopic margin involvement [74].

Regional lymph node metastasis is the other important determinant of prognosis after distant metastasis. Lymph node involvement is alone an indication for post-operative adjuvant therapy to reduce the metastasis risk. Although the number of positive lymph nodes involved is a crucial predictor of outcome [74, 88], relationship between total number of the lymph nodes and the prognosis is not well understood. However, increased number of total lymph nodes in the surgical specimen may be an indicator for the quality of the surgical procedure [88].

Tumor deposits are separate nodules of tumor within the pericolic fat or mesentery. In the TNM staging they are staged as N1c which means there are no regional lymph nodes involved but the subserosa, mesentery, or nonperitonealized pericolic tissues contains tumor deposits(74). These deposits are strong adverse prognostic determinants, and there is a relation between extramural extranodal tumor deposits and extramural venous invasion [89, 90]. Lymphovascular involvement which is tumor invasion into veins, especially extramural veins, or lymphatics is thought to be an adverse prognostic factor [91–93]. Perineural invasion is also associated with an elevated risk of recurrence and poor prognosis [94, 95].

Several studies have provided evidence that preoperative high CEA levels have adverse impact on prognosis for colon cancer. It has been determined that higher CEA levels increase overall mortality and even prognosis is similar or worse in patients with higher CEA levels but lower stages when compared to patients with higher stages but lower CEA levels according to AJCC TNM staging [96, 97].

Metastatic disease is another significant clinical problem in patients with CRCs. The liver, lungs, lymph nodes, and peritoneum are the most frequently involved organs. Major developments in chemotherapy have increased survival rates in a serious manner, but 5-year survival rates are below 20% without resection or ablation of metastasis. Five-year survival rates are 36–58% in patients undergoing partial hepatectomy for hepatic metastases [98–102]. Lung involvement is less common than liver metastasis, but in carefully selected patients metastasectomy is a favorable option for treatment [102].

Conflict of interest

The authors declare that there are no conflicts of interest.

DOI: http://dx.doi.org/10.5772/intechopen.81597

Author details

Mehmet Ali Koc[1], Suleyman Utku Celik[2] and Cihangir Akyol[1]*

1 Department of General Surgery, Ankara University School of Medicine, Ankara, Turkey

2 Clinic of General Surgery, Gulhane Training and Research Hospital, Ankara, Turkey

*Address all correspondence to: cihangirakyol@gmail.com

References

[1] Torre LA, Bray F, Siegel RL, et al. Global cancer statistics, 2012. CA: A Cancer Journal for Clinicians. 2015;**65**(2):87-108

[2] Howlader N, Noone AM, Krapcho M, et al. SEER Cancer Statistics Review (CSR) 1975-2014. https://seer.cancer.gov/archive/csr/1975_2014/

[3] Gordon PH. Malignant neoplasms of the colon. In: Gordon PH, Nivatvongs S, editors. Principles and Practice of Surgery for the Colon; Rectum; and Anus. 3rd ed. New York: Informa Healthcare USA Inc.; 2007. pp. 489-643

[4] Ryan-Harshman M, Aldoori W. Diet and colorectal cancer: Review of the evidence. Canadian Family Physician. 2007;**53**(11):1913-1920

[5] Akin H, Tözün N. Diet, microbiota, and colorectal cancer. Journal of Clinical Gastroenterology. 2014;**48**(Suppl 1): S67-S69

[6] Itzkowitz SH, Rochester J. Colonic polyps and polyposis syndromes. In: Feldman M, Fiedman LS, Brandt LJ, editors. Gastrointestinal and Liver Disease. 8th ed. Philadelphia: Saunders Elsevier; 2006. pp. 2713-2757

[7] Calle EE, Rodriguez C, Walker-Thurmond K, et al. Overweight, obesity, and mortality from cancer in a prospectively studied cohort of U.S. adults. The New England Journal of Medicine. 2003;**348**(17):1625-1638

[8] Kim ER, Chang DK. Colorectal cancer in inflammatory bowel disease: The risk, pathogenesis, prevention and diagnosis. World Journal of Gastroenterology. 2014;**20**(29):9872-9881

[9] Eaden JA. The risk of colorectal cancer in ulcerative colitis: A meta-analysis. Gut. 2001;**48**(4):526-535

[10] Shergill AK, Farraye FA. Toward a consensus on endoscopic surveillance of patients with colonic inflammatory bowel disease. Gastrointestinal Endoscopy Clinics of North America. 2014;**24**(3):469-481

[11] Zauber AG, Winawer SJ, O'Brien MJ, et al. Colonoscopic polypectomy and long-term prevention of colorectal-cancer deaths. The New England Journal of Medicine. 2012;**366**(8):687-696

[12] Grady WM, Markowitz SD. The molecular pathogenesis of colorectal cancer and its potential application to colorectal cancer screening. Digestive Diseases and Sciences. 2015;**60**(3):762-772

[13] Grady WM, Carethers JM. Genomic and epigenetic instability in colorectal cancer pathogenesis. Gastroenterology. 2008;**135**(4):1079-1099

[14] Vogelstein B, Fearon ER, Hamilton SR, et al. Genetic alterations during colorectal-tumor development. The New England Journal of Medicine. 1988;**319**(9):525-532

[15] Fodde R. The APC gene in colorectal cancer. European Journal of Cancer. 2002;**38**(7):867-871

[16] Powell SM, Zilz N, Beazer-Barclay Y, et al. APC mutations occur early during colorectal tumorigenesis. Nature. **359**(6392):235-237

[17] Cancer Genome Atlas Network. Comprehensive molecular characterization of human colon and rectal cancer. Nature. 2012;**487**(7407):330-337

[18] Hedrick L, Cho KR, Fearon ER, Wu TC, Kinzler KW, Vogelstein B. The DCC gene product in cellular differentiation and colorectal tumorigenesis. Genes & Development. 1994;**8**(10):1174-1183

[19] Xie W, Rimm DL, Lin Y, Shih WJ, Reiss M. Loss of Smad signaling in human colorectal cancer is associated with advanced disease and poor prognosis. Cancer Journal. 2003;**9**(4):302-312

[20] Martín M, Simon-Assmann P, Kedinger M, Martin M, Mangeat P, Real FX, et al. DCC regulates cell adhesion in human colon cancer derived HT-29 cells and associates with ezrin. European Journal of Cell Biology. 2006;**85**(8):769-783

[21] Kuerbitz SJ, Plunkett BS, Walsh WV, Kastan MB. Wild-type p53 is a cell cycle checkpoint determinant following irradiation. Proceedings of the National Academy of Sciences of the United States of America. 1992;**89**(16):7491-7495

[22] Fearon ER, Vogelstein B. A genetic model for colorectal tumorigenesis. Cell. 1990;**61**(5):759-767

[23] Bahnassy AA, Zekri AR, Salem SE, et al. Differential expression of p53 family proteins in colorectal adenomas and carcinomas: Prognostic and predictive values. Histology and Histopathology. 2014;**29**(2):207-216

[24] Söreide K, Janssen EA, Söiland H, Körner H, Baak JP. Microsatellite instability in colorectal cancer. The British Journal of Surgery. 2006;**93**(4):395-406

[25] Jones PA, Laird PW. Cancer epigenetics comes of age. Nature Genetics. 1999;**21**(2):163-167

[26] Baylin SB, Herman JG. DNA hypermethylation in tumorigenesis: Epigenetics joins genetics. Trends in Genetics. 2000;**16**(4):168-174

[27] Herman JG, Umar A, Polyak K, et al. Incidence and functional consequences of hMLH1 promoter hypermethylation in colorectal carcinoma. Proceedings of the National Academy of Sciences of the United States of America. 1998;**95**(12):6870-6875

[28] Domingo E, Niessen RC, Oliveira C, et al. BRAF-V600E is not involved in the colorectal tumorigenesis of HNPCC in patients with functional MLH1 and MSH2 genes. Oncogene. 2005;**24**(24):3995-3998

[29] Rajagopalan H, Bardelli A, Lengauer C, et al. Tumorigenesis: RAF/RAS oncogenes and mismatch-repair status. Nature. 2002;**418**(6901):934

[30] Moreira L, Balaguer F, Lindor N, et al. Identification of Lynch syndrome among patients with colorectal cancer. JAMA. 2012;**308**(15):1555-1565

[31] Win AK, Buchanan DD, Rosty C, et al. Role of tumour molecular and pathology features to estimate colorectal cancer risk for first-degree relatives. Gut. 2015;**64**(1):101-110

[32] Parry S, Win AK, Parry B, et al. Metachronous colorectal cancer risk for mismatch repair gene mutation carriers: The advantage of more extensive colon surgery. Gut. 2011;**60**(7):950-957

[33] Møller P, Seppälä T, Bernstein I, et al. Incidence of and survival after subsequent cancers in carriers of pathogenic MMR variants with previous cancer: A report from the prospective Lynch syndrome database. Gut. 2017;**66**(9):1657-1664

[34] Umar A, Boland CR, Terdiman JP, et al. Revised Bethesda guidelines for hereditary nonpolyposis colorectal cancer (Lynch syndrome) and microsatellite instability. Journal of the National Cancer Institute. 2004;**96**(4):261-268

[35] Vasen H, Watson P, Mecklin J, et al. New clinical criteria for hereditary nonpolyposis colorectal cancer (HNPCC, Lynch syndrome) proposed

by the International Collaborative group on HNPCC. Gastroenterology. 1999;**116**(6):1453-1456

[36] Syngal S, Brand RE, Church JM, et al. ACG clinical guideline: Genetic testing and management of hereditary gastrointestinal cancer syndromes. The American Journal of Gastroenterology. 2015;**110**(2):223-262; quiz 263

[37] Giardiello FM, Allen JI, Axilbund JE, et al. Guidelines on genetic evaluation and management of Lynch syndrome: A consensus statement by the US multi-society task force on colorectal cancer. Gastroenterology. 2014;**147**(2):502-526

[38] Win AK, Parry S, Parry B, et al. Risk of metachronous colon cancer following surgery for rectal cancer in mismatch repair gene mutation carriers. Annals of Surgical Oncology. 2013;**20**(6):1829-1836

[39] Kalady MF, McGannon E, Vogel JD, et al. Risk of colorectal adenoma and carcinoma after colectomy for colorectal cancer in patients meeting Amsterdam criteria. Annals of Surgery. 2010;**252**(3):507-511

[40] Burt RW, DiSario JA, Cannon-Albright L. Genetics of colon cancer: Impact of inheritance on colon cancer risk. Annual Review of Medicine. 1995;**46**:371-379

[41] Hernegger GS, Moore HG, Guillem JG. Attenuated familial adenomatous polyposis: An evolving and poorly understood entity. Diseases of the Colon and Rectum. 2002;**45**(1):127-134; discussion 134-6

[42] Lamlum H, Papadopoulou A, Ilyas M, et al. APC mutations are sufficient for the growth of early colorectal adenomas. Proceedings of the National Academy of Sciences of the United States of America. 2000;**97**(5):2225-2228

[43] Burt RW. Gastric fundic gland polyps. Gastroenterology. 2003;**125**(5):1462-1469

[44] Wallace MH, Phillips RK. Upper gastrointestinal disease in patients with familial adenomatous polyposis. The British Journal of Surgery. 1998;**85**(6):742-750

[45] Jagelman DG, DeCosse JJ, Bussey HJ. Upper gastrointestinal cancer in familial adenomatous polyposis. Lancet. 1988;**1**(8595):1149-1151

[46] Church J, Xhaja X, Laguardia L, et al. Desmoids and genotype in familial adenomatous polyposis. Diseases of the Colon and Rectum. 2015;**58**(4):444-448

[47] Soravia C, Berk T, McLeod RS, et al. Desmoid disease in patients with familial adenomatous polyposis. Diseases of the Colon and Rectum. 2000;**43**(3):363-369

[48] Clark SK, Neale KF, Landgrebe JC, et al. Desmoid tumours complicating familial adenomatous polyposis. The British Journal of Surgery. 1999;**86**(9):1185-1189

[49] Robinson WA, McMillan C, Kendall A, et al. Desmoid tumors in pregnant and postpartum women. Cancers (Basel). 2012;**4**(1):184-192

[50] Nieuwenhuis MH, Lefevre JH, Bülow S, et al. Family history, surgery, and APC mutation are risk factors for desmoid tumors in familial adenomatous polyposis: An international cohort study. Diseases of the Colon and Rectum. 2011;**54**(10):1229-1234

[51] Touriño R, Conde-Freire R, Cabezas-Agrícola JM, et al. Value of the congenital hypertrophy of the retinal pigment epithelium in the diagnosis of familial adenomatous polyposis. International Ophthalmology. 2004;**25**(2):101-112

[52] Sener SF, Miller HH, Decosse JJ. The spectrum of polyposis. Surgery, Gynecology & Obstetrics. 1984;**159**(6):525-532

[53] Itoh H, Hirata K, Ohsato K. Turcot's syndrome and familial adenomatous polyposis associated with brain tumor: Review of related literature. International Journal of Colorectal Disease. 1993;**8**(2):87-94

[54] Vasen HFA, Moslein G, Alonso A, et al. Guidelines for the clinical management of familial adenomatous polyposis (FAP). Gut. 2008;**57**(5):704-713

[55] Jarrar AM, Milas M, Mitchell J, et al. Screening for thyroid cancer in patients with familial adenomatous polyposis. Annals of Surgery. 2011;**253**(3):515-521

[56] Feng X, Milas M, O'Malley M, et al. Characteristics of benign and malignant thyroid disease in familial adenomatous polyposis patients and recommendations for disease surveillance. Thyroid. 2015;**25**(3):325-332

[57] Cruz-Correa M, Hylind LM, Romans KE, Booker SV, Giardiello FM. Long-term treatment with sulindac in familial adenomatous polyposis: A prospective cohort study. Gastroenterology. 2002;**122**(3):641-645

[58] Lynch PM, Ayers GD, Hawk E, et al. The safety and efficacy of celecoxib in children with familial adenomatous polyposis. The American Journal of Gastroenterology. 2010;**105**(6):1437-1443

[59] Winawer SJ, Zauber AG, Gerdes H, et al. Risk of colorectal cancer in the families of patients with adenomatous polyps. National Polyp Study Workgroup. The New England Journal of Medicine. 1996;**334**(2):82-87

[60] Johns LE, Houlston RS. A systematic review and meta-analysis of familial colorectal cancer risk. The American Journal of Gastroenterology. 2001;**96**(10):2992-3003

[61] Church J. Ileoanal pouch neoplasia in familial adenomatous polyposis: An underestimated threat. Diseases of the Colon and Rectum. 2005;**48**(9):1708-1713

[62] Sieber OM, Lipton L, Crabtree M, et al. Multiple colorectal adenomas, classic adenomatous polyposis, and germ-line mutations in MYH. The New England Journal of Medicine. 2003;**348**(9):791-799

[63] Grover S, Kastrinos F, Steyerberg EW, et al. Prevalence and phenotypes of APC and MUTYH mutations in patients with multiple colorectal adenomas. JAMA. 2012;**308**(5):485-492

[64] Win AK, Dowty JG, Cleary SP, et al. Risk of colorectal cancer for carriers of mutations in MUTYH, with and without a family history of cancer. Gastroenterology. 2014;**146**(5):1208-1211

[65] Moreno CC, Mittal PK, Sullivan PS, et al. Colorectal cancer initial diagnosis: Screening colonoscopy, diagnostic colonoscopy, or emergent surgery, and tumor stage and size at initial presentation. Clinical Colorectal Cancer. 2016;**15**(1):67-73

[66] Hamilton W, Round A, Sharp D, et al. Clinical features of colorectal cancer before diagnosis: A population-based case-control study. British Journal of Cancer. 2005;**93**(4):399-405

[67] Thompson MR, O'Leary DP, Flashman K, et al. Clinical assessment to determine the risk of bowel cancer using Symptoms, Age, Mass and Iron deficiency anaemia (SAMI). The British Journal of Surgery. 2017;**104**(10):1393-1404

[68] Chang GJ, Kaiser AM, Mills S, et al. Practice parameters for the management

of colon cancer. Diseases of the Colon and Rectum. 2012;**55**(8):831-843

[69] Goodman D, Irvin TT. Delay in the diagnosis and prognosis of carcinoma of the right colon. The British Journal of Surgery. 1993;**80**(10):1327-1329

[70] Siegel RL, Miller KD, Jemal A. Cancer statistics, 2016. CA: A Cancer Journal for Clinicians. 2016;**66**(1):7-30

[71] Mulder SA, Kranse R, Damhuis RA, et al. Prevalence and prognosis of synchronous colorectal cancer: A Dutch population-based study. Cancer Epidemiology. 2011;**35**(5):442-447

[72] Passman MA, Pommier RF, Vetto JT. Synchronous colon primaries have the same prognosis as solitary colon cancers. Diseases of the Colon and Rectum. 1996;**39**(3):329-334

[73] Liu Z, Zhang Y, Niu Y, et al. A systematic review and meta-analysis of diagnostic and prognostic serum biomarkers of colorectal cancer. PLoS One. 2014;**9**(8):e103910

[74] Jesssup JM, Goldberg RM, Aware EA, et al. Colon and rectum. In: Amin M, editor. AJCC Cancer Staging Manual. 8th ed. Chicago; 2017. p. 251

[75] Hohenberger W, Merkel S, Weber K. Lymphadenektomie bei tumoren des unteren gastrointestinaltraktes. Chirurg. 2007;**78**(3):217-225

[76] Hohenberger W, Weber K, Matzel K, et al. Standardized surgery for colonic cancer: Complete mesocolic excision and central ligation-technical notes and outcome. Colorectal Disease. 2009 May;**11**(4):354-364; discussion 364-5

[77] West NP, Hohenberger W, Weber K, et al. Complete mesocolic excision with central vascular ligation produces an oncologically superior specimen compared with standard surgery for carcinoma of the colon. Journal of Clinical Oncology. 2010;**28**(2):272-278

[78] Galizia G, Lieto E, De Vita F, et al. Is complete mesocolic excision with central vascular ligation safe and effective in the surgical treatment of right-sided colon cancers? A prospective study. International Journal of Colorectal Disease. 2014;**29**(1):89-97

[79] Bertelsen CA, Bols B, Ingeholm P, et al. Can the quality of colonic surgery be improved by standardization of surgical technique with complete mesocolic excision? Colorectal Disease. 2011;**13**(10):1123-1129

[80] Feng B, Sun J, Ling TL, et al. Laparoscopic complete mesocolic excision (CME) with medial access for right-hemi colon cancer: Feasibility and technical strategies. Surgical Endoscopy. 2012;**26**(12):3669-3675

[81] Renouf DJ, Woods R, Speers C, et al. Improvements in 5-year outcomes of stage II/III rectal cancer relative to colon cancer. American Journal of Clinical Oncology. 2013;**36**(6):558-564

[82] Sargent D, Sobrero A, Grothey A, et al. Evidence for cure by adjuvant therapy in colon cancer: Observations based on individual patient data from 20,898 patients on 18 randomized trials. Journal of Clinical Oncology. 2009;**27**(6):872-877

[83] Shepherd NA, Baxter KJ, Love SB. The prognostic importance of peritoneal involvement in colonic cancer: A prospective evaluation. Gastroenterology;**112**(4):1096-1102

[84] Chapuis PH, Dent OF, Fisher R, et al. A multivariate analysis of clinical and pathological variables in prognosis after resection of large bowel cancer. The British Journal of Surgery. 1985;**72**(9):698-702

[85] Newland RCC, Dent OFF, Lyttle MNN, et al. Pathologic determinants

of survival associated with colorectal cancer with lymph node metastases. A multivariate analysis of 579 patients. Cancer. 1994;**73**(8):2076-2082

[86] Wittekind C, Compton CC, Greene FL, et al. TNM residual tumor classification revisited. Cancer. 2002;**94**(9):2511-2516

[87] Compton C, Fenoglio-Preiser CM, Pettigrew N, Fielding LP. American Joint Committee on Cancer Prognostic Factors Consensus Conference: Colorectal Working Group. Cancer. 2000;**88**(7):1739-1757

[88] Chen SL, Bilchik AJ. More extensive nodal dissection improves survival for stages I to III of colon cancer: A population-based study. Annals of Surgery. 2006;**244**(4):602-610

[89] Goldstein NS, Turner JR. Pericolonic tumor deposits in patients with T3N+M0 colon adenocarcinomas: Markers of reduced disease free survival and intra-abdominal metastases and their implications for TNM classification. Cancer. 2000;**88**(10):2228-2238

[90] Lord AC, D'Souza N, Pucher PH, et al. Significance of extranodal tumour deposits in colorectal cancer: A systematic review and meta-analysis. European Journal of Cancer. 2017;**82**:92-102

[91] Siddiqui MRS, Simillis C, Hunter C, et al. A meta-analysis comparing the risk of metastases in patients with rectal cancer and MRI-detected extramural vascular invasion (mrEMVI) vs mrEMVI-negative cases. British Journal of Cancer. 2017;**116**(12):1513-1519

[92] Lim SB, Yu CS, Jang SJ, et al. Prognostic significance of lymphovascular invasion in sporadic colorectal cancer. Diseases of the Colon and Rectum. 2010;**53**(4):377-384

[93] Betge J, Pollheimer MJ, Lindtner RA, et al. Intramural and extramural vascular invasion in colorectal cancer: Prognostic significance and quality of pathology reporting. Cancer. 2012;**118**(3):628-638

[94] Huh JW, Kim HR, Kim YJ. Prognostic value of perineural invasion in patients with stage II colorectal cancer. Annals of Surgical Oncology. 2010;**17**(8):2066-2072

[95] Liebig C, Ayala G, Wilks J, et al. Perineural invasion is an independent predictor of outcome in colorectal cancer. Journal of Clinical Oncology. 2009;**27**(31):5131-5137

[96] Thirunavukarasu P, Sukumar S, Sathaiah M, et al. C-stage in colon cancer: Implications of carcinoembryonic antigen biomarker in staging, prognosis, and management. Journal of the National Cancer Institute. 2011;**103**(8):689-697

[97] Thirunavukarasu P, Talati C, Munjal S, et al. Effect of incorporation of pretreatment serum carcinoembryonic antigen levels into AJCC staging for colon cancer on 5-year survival. JAMA Surgery. 2015;**150**(8):747-755

[98] Morris EJA, Forman D, Thomas JD, et al. Surgical management and outcomes of colorectal cancer liver metastases. The British Journal of Surgery. 2010;**97**(7):1110-1118

[99] De Jong MC, Pulitano C, Ribero D, et al. Rates and patterns of recurrence following curative intent surgery for colorectal liver metastasis: An international multi-institutional analysis of 1669 patients. Annals of Surgery. 2009;**250**(3):440-447

[100] Rees M, Tekkis PP, Welsh FKS, et al. Evaluation of long-term survival after hepatic resection for metastatic colorectal cancer: A multifactorial model of 929 patients. Annals of Surgery. 2008;**247**(1):125-135

[101] Wei AC, Greig PD, Grant D, et al. Survival after hepatic resection for colorectal metastases: A 10-year experience. Annals of Surgical Oncology. 2006;**13**(5):668-676

[102] Abdalla EK, Vauthey JN, Ellis LM, et al. Recurrence and outcomes following hepatic resection, radiofrequency ablation, and combined resection/ablation for colorectal liver metastases. Annals of Surgery. 2004;**239**(6):818-825

Section 3

Urogenital Cancers

Chapter 5

Exploring New Molecular Targets in Advanced Ovarian Cancer: The Aryl Hydrocarbon Receptor (AhR) and Antitumor Benzothiazole Ligands as Potential Therapeutic Candidates

Andrea I. Loaiza Perez and Tracey D. Bradshaw

Abstract

Antitumor benzothiazoles, including 2-(4-amino-3-methylphenyl)-5-fluoro-benzothiazole (5F 203; NSC 703786), non-fluorinated parent compound DF 203 (NSC 674495), and Phortress (NSC 710305), the lysyl amide prodrug of 5F 203, are experimental anticancer agents with activity in ovarian and breast cancer models *in vitro* and *in vivo*. These compounds require (and induce their own) metabolism by cytochrome P450 (CYP) enzymes (e.g., CYP1A1) for antitumor action. The aryl hydrocarbon receptor (AhR) is the main transcriptional regulator of CYP1A1, and we have previously demonstrated that DF 203 and 5F 203 are potent AhR ligands and trigger activation of AhR signaling in sensitive breast and ovarian cancer cells, causing nuclear translocation of AhR. We propose that AhR may represent a new molecular target in the treatment of ovarian tumors, and 5F 203 may exemplify a potential novel treatment. Furthermore, putative biomarkers of sensitivity to this agent have been identified.

Keywords: ovarian cancer, AhR, benzothiazoles

1. Introduction

Ovarian cancer is one of the most lethal gynecological cancers. The National Cancer Institute (NCI) estimated ~22,240 new cases with ~14,070 deaths from ovarian cancer in the US in 2018 [1]. Globally, in 2012, 239,000 women were diagnosed with ovarian carcinoma and 152,000 deaths from this disease were recorded [2]. Unfortunately, the majority of cases are only diagnosed at advanced stages (stage III or IV), a consequence of the cancer's asymptomatic nature, and overall survival lies between 5 and 25% [3, 4]. Hence, the inability to detect this disease during early stages has led to poor prognosis. Despite improvements in medicine and patient care, screening for detection of early-stage ovarian cancer is presently lacking. Thus, a better understanding of the molecular events that underlie ovarian cancer development is needed.

IntechOpen

The current strategy for treatment of ovarian cancer is surgery followed by radiotherapy and chemotherapy [3, 4]. Although ~70% of ovarian cancer patients respond initially to a combination of platinum and taxane-based chemotherapy, drug-resistance emerges and current treatments are of limited efficacy in preventing tumor recurrence and progression [3, 4]. Thus, despite surgery, radiotherapy, and chemotherapy, most patients present with recurrent disease within 12–18 months, which spreads rapidly within the peritoneal cavity. In platinum-resistant disease, survival rarely exceeds 5 months [1, 5]. Thus, new anti-neoplastic agents are urgently needed to improve the prognoses for ovarian cancer patients. Recently, evidence has emerged revealing the importance of genomic aberrations in the progression of ovarian cancer [6–8]. Through the use of high-throughput technologies (i.e., array comparative genomic hybridization (aCGH), microarray, and SNP arrays), specific genomic regions have been identified to be either amplified or silenced in tumor progression [6, 7].

Molecularly targeted cancer therapies recently introduced into the clinic include drugs designed to interfere with specific proteins ("molecular targets") that are involved in the growth, progression, and spread of cancer. Used in the treatment of ovarian cancer are bevacizumab (a VEGF inhibitor) [9], olaparib [10], and niraparib (PARP inhibitors) [11].

The objective of our work has been for many years to validate the aryl hydrocarbon receptor as a molecular target of antitumor drugs, for the treatment of different cancers including ovarian cancer.

1.1 The aryl hydrocarbon receptor as a putative molecular target for cancer therapeutics

1.1.1 AhR structure

The aryl hydrocarbon receptor (AhR) was initially defined as a receptor for environmental toxins such as dioxin. It has been described as a "pioneer member" of the basic-helix/loop/helix PER-ARNT-SIM (bHLH/PAS) family of "sensors" of foreign and endogenous signals [12].

As intimated, other members include AhR nuclear translocator (ARNT); *drosophila* proteins, single-minded (SIM) and period (PER); and hypoxia inducible factor 1α (HIF 1α) [13–16]. AhR is a ligand-activated transcription factor. The most commonly known ligands of AhR are polycyclic and polyhalogenated hydrocarbons (benzopyrene, 3-methyl-colanthrene), xenobiotics (phenobarbital), and other pesticides such as tetrachlorodibenzo-p-dioxin (TCDD).

1.1.2 AhR activation and signaling

AhR is localized within the cell cytosol constitutively where it is part of an inactivated complex composed of two heat-shock proteins: heat-shock protein 90 (Hsp90), the aryl hydrocarbon receptor interacting protein (AIP), and a 23-kDa protein (p23) (**Figure 1**). Hsp90 acts as a chaperone maintaining AhR in a favorable ligand-binding configuration while preventing its nuclear translocation. Hydrophobic ligands of AhR enter the cell by diffusion and bind to the receptor associated to Hsp90. Ligand binding to the receptor triggers a conformational change in AhR to a form that exhibits stronger affinity for DNA. This event leads to dissociation of the cytoplasmic complex and AhR nuclear translocation. In the nucleus, AhR interacts with ARNT forming a heterodimer that binds to specific DNA sequences—the xenobiotic response elements (XREs) in the promoter regions of genes within the AhR gene battery. Binding leads to transcriptional activation of

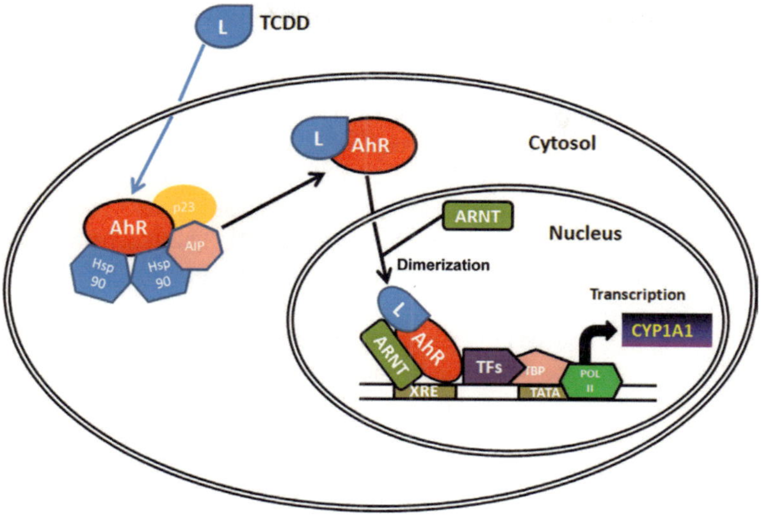

Figure 1.
The aryl hydrocarbon receptor signaling pathway.

genes activated by AhR including those encoding phase I and II metabolic enzymes such as cytochrome P450 (CYP) 1A1, CYP1A2, and CYP1B1. AhR activation was first described as a cellular response to promote elimination of ambient contaminants and xenobiotics [17–19]. In humans, AhR is localized in liver, lungs, kidneys, placenta, lymphocytes, ovary, and breast. AhR/ARNT complex activation is tissue-specific and depends on co-regulators and repressors present in different cell types [18].

1.2 The importance of AhR in ovarian cancer

Functional AhR has been reported in rat and mouse uteri. AhR knockout mice exhibited no histopathological changes in uterine tissues; however, dioxin inhibited estrogen-induced responses including estrogen receptor (ER) binding in rat uteri. In addition, *in utero* and lactational exposure to dioxin results in decreased uterine weights in female offspring during estrus and diestrus. The female reproductive tract expresses mRNA for the transcription factors AhR and ARNT, and changes in their expression at select target sites in specific pathological conditions such as endometriosis and uterine leiomyomas suggest a potential role for these factors in the pathogenesis of these conditions [20].

The role of the AhR and AhR agonists has not been extensively investigated in endometrial and ovarian cancer cell lines; however, there is evidence that AhR-ERα cross talk and growth inhibitory pathways are operative [21–23], requiring further investigation.

Intriguingly, immune suppression in ovarian cancer has been described, with a particular focus on the potential involvement of the c-KIT/PI3K/AKT, wnt/β-catenin, IL-6/STAT3, and AhR signaling pathways in regulation of indoleamine 2,3-dioxygenase expression in tumor-associated macrophages [24].

AhR has important roles in homeostasis and evidence is accumulating to support its contribution to disease pathogenesis—including cancer. AhR expression has been detected in multiple tumor types and its function probed by RNA interference, over-expression, and inhibition studies. AhR knockdown led to decreased cancer cell proliferation, migration, and invasion *in vitro*, and *in vivo*, constitutive over-expression resulted in enhanced stomach and liver cancers, suggesting a pro-oncogenic role. In contrast, loss of AhR in transgenic mice that spontaneously develop colorectal carcinoma (CRC) and carcinogen-induced tumors led to increased carcinogenesis suggesting a tumor-suppressive role for AhR [25].

Specific to this review, AhR has been found to be widely expressed in many histotypes of ovarian cancer tissue; in the ovarian cancer tissue microarray, the AhR immunoreactivity was present in disgerminoma (DISG), adenocarcinoma (ADEN), teratoma malignant change (TMC), yolk sac tumor (YST), mucinous adenocarcinoma (Mu-ADEN), serous adenocarcinoma (low grade (L-Se-ADEN) and high grade (H-Se-ADEN), but not in normal tissue (NORM). The semi-quantification analysis revealed that the value in NORM was similar to that in DISG and ADEN, but was much lower than that in TMC, YST, Mu-ADEN, and L- and H-Se-ADEN. No difference was detected between the grades, stages, and tumor node metastasis classifications in each histotype of ovarian cancer tissues studied. Moreover, the endogenous AhR ligand 2-(1′H-indole-3′-carbonyl)-thiazole-4-carboxylic acid methyl ester (ITE) inhibited proliferation of OVCAR-3 cells and migration of SKOV-3 cells *in vitro* and suppressed growth of OVCAR-3 cell xenografts in mice [26].

1.3 Benzothiazoles and aminoflavone: AhR-targeted anticancer therapies

The benzothiazole (Bz) class of experimental antitumor agent includes 2-(4-amino-3-methylphenyl)-5-fluorobenzothiazole (5F 203; NSC 703786; **Figure 2**); non-fluorinated parent compound DF 203 (NSC 674495); and Phortress (NSC 710305), the lysyl amide prodrug of 5F 203. These experimental antitumor agents elicit potent and selective antitumor activity *in vitro* against certain cell lines originating from breast (irrespective of ER status) and ovarian carcinomas. Empirical screening in the NCI cell line anticancer drug screen revealed that the Bzs [27–32] and also aminoflavone (AF) [33] were noteworthy for their distinct (selective and potent) patterns of growth inhibitory activity. "Sensitive" cell lines caused total carcinoma cell growth inhibition (TGI) between 0.1 and 1 μM, while "resistant" cell lines are refractory to Bz and AF (TGI concentrations <10 μM). Among the consistently sensitive cell lines to both compound classes were the ER (+) breast cancer cell lines MCF-7 and T47D, certain ovarian (e.g., IGROV-1) and renal (TK10) cancer cell lines [34]. Intriguingly, IGROV-1 cells developed in the laboratory possessing acquired resistance to cisplatin were equi-sensitive to antitumor Bzs as IGROV-1 parental cells. Detailed mechanistic studies for both Bzs and AF identified a mode of action distinct from current clinical chemotherapeutic agents. In "sensitive" cells, Bzs and AF activate AhR signaling, as might be anticipated from their planar structures [35].

AhR signal transduction induces expression of CYP1A1 and (in certain cell lines) CYP1B1. Prior work has demonstrated that CYP1A1 can metabolize (actively biotransform) Bzs and AF to produce DNA-damaging metabolites [30, 33] (**Figure 2**). For example, DNA adducts, single- and double-strand breaks have been detected exclusively in sensitive cells exposed to 2-(4-amino-3-methylphenyl)-5-fluorobenzothiazole (5F 203), and in Bz-sensitive tumor xenografts extracted from Phortress-treated mice [36–39]. Subsequently, it was irrefutably demonstrated that CYP1A1-bioactivation of 5F 203 resulted in generation of an electrophilic species (nitrenium ion) able to form glutathione conjugates and dGuo adducts [40].

1.4 5F 203 activity in ovarian cancer

Antitumor Bzs, including 2-(4-amino-3-methylphenyl)-5-fluorobenzothiazole (5F 203; NSC 703786; **Figure 2**), non-fluorinated parent compound DF 203 (NSC 674495), and Phortress (NSC 710305), the lysyl amide prodrug of 5F 203, are experimental anticancer agents with activity in ovarian and breast cancer models *in vitro* and *in vivo* (**Figure 3A** and **B**) [36, 41].

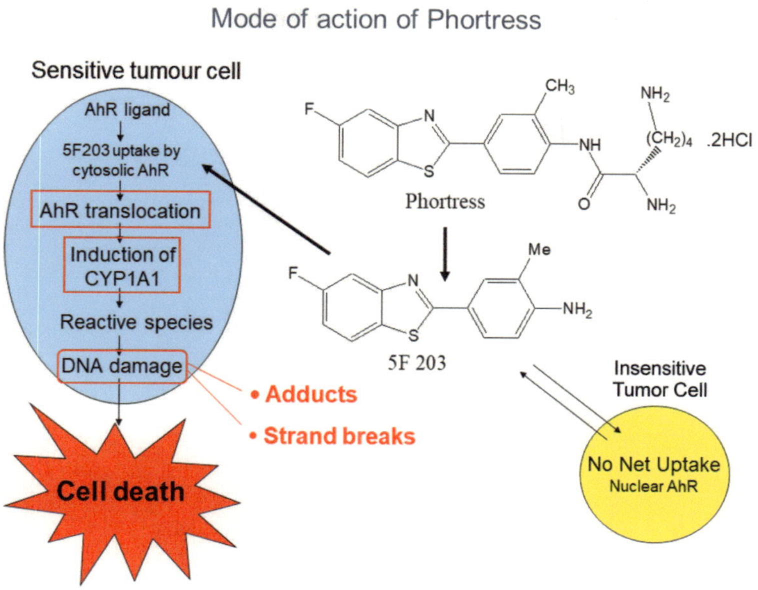

Figure 2.
5F 203, liberated from Phortress binds cytosolic AhR, triggering nuclear translocation and binding to the XRE within the promoter region of AhR-battery genes including CYP 1A1. This enzyme-catalyzed biotransformation of 5F 203 produces nitrenium species that generate lethal DNA adducts at nucleophilic sites precipitating DNA double-strand breaks and apoptosis, exclusively in sensitive cells. In inherently resistant cells, there is no net cellular uptake of lipophilic 5F 203.

As introduced, these compounds require metabolism by cytochrome P450 (CYP) enzymes (e.g., CYP1A1) for antitumor action. The aryl hydrocarbon receptor (AhR) is the main transcriptional regulator of CYP1A1 and we have previously demonstrated that DF 203 and 5F 203 induce activation of AhR signaling in sensitive breast cancer cells, causing nuclear translocation of AhR [27–29]. Also, IGROV-1 human ovarian cancer cells, sensitive to 5F 203 treatment, show induction of CYP1A1 expression by 5F 203 and Phortress (**Figure 3B**), whereas SKOV-3 cells, resistant to these agents, express neither constitutive nor inducible CYP1A1 [42]. Fine needle aspirates obtained from IGROV-1 human xenografts, treated *ex vivo* with 5F 203, resulted in induction of CYP1A1 expression. This was not observed in 5F 203-resistant tumors. It was proposed that induction of *cyp1a1* mRNA in response to 5F 203 treatment *ex vivo* might provide a possible biomarker for determination of drug-sensitive ovarian tumors in patients [42]. Compounds that activate AhR signaling and induce CYP expression frequently generate reactive oxygen species (ROS) in susceptible cells.

Experimental and clinical evidence has emerged linking oxidative stress to pathologies including carcinogenesis [43]. However, oxidative stress is not always detrimental, and may, if induced in a selective manner, be of therapeutic benefit. Many chemotherapeutic agents induce oxidative stress integral to their antitumor mechanism [44]. High-grade ovarian tumors generally present high ROS levels and respond better to treatment with antitumor agents that induce further ROS, such as paclitaxel [45]. In addition, c-JUN amino terminal kinase (JNK), ERK, and P38MAPK sustained activation have key roles in cellular stress-induced apoptosis [46].

1.5 5F 203 induces AhR translocation and activation of CYP 1A1-related promoter sequences in 5F 203-sensitive ovarian cancer cells

It has been established that 5F 203 is a potent AhR ligand [35] able to induce nuclear translocation of AhR with subsequent binding to XRE sequences resulting

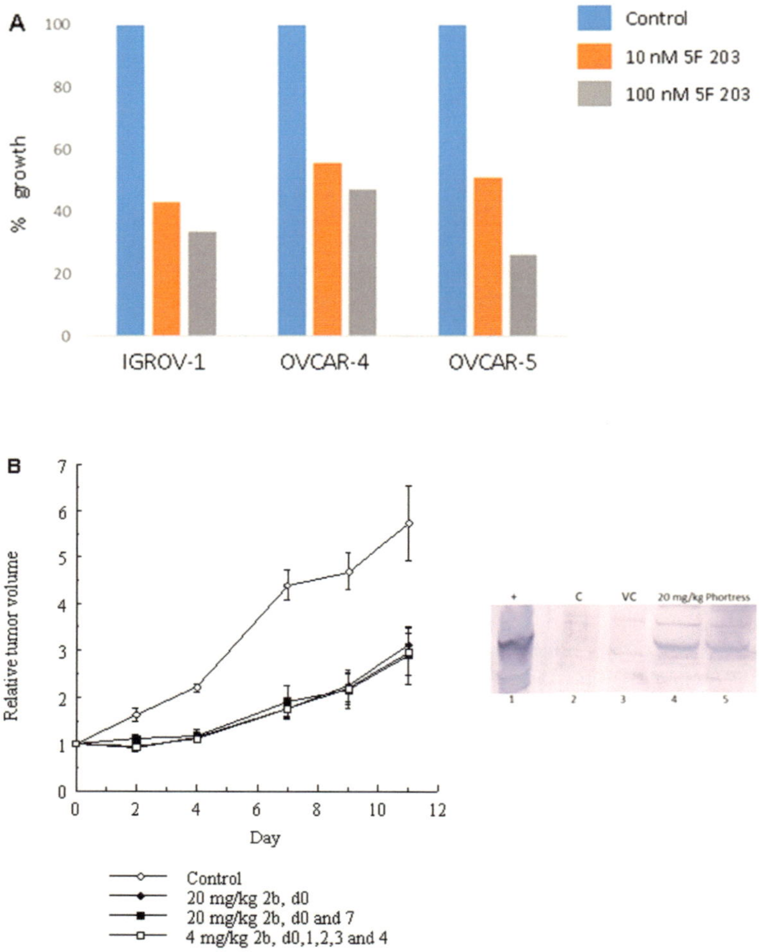

Figure 3.
A. In vitro growth inhibitory activity of 5F 203 against ovarian carcinoma cell lines. Representative data generated at the NCI are shown. Cells were exposed to test agent for 48 h before growth was assessed by sulforhodamine blue (SRB) assay. B. In vivo Phortress efficacy against IGROV-1 ovarian tumor xenografts. IGROV-1 ovarian xenografts were transplanted s.c. into flanks of NCR-Nu female nude mice. Animals were treated i.v. with Phortress in saline according to the indicated schedules. Control animals received vehicle alone. Tumor volumes were measured using calipers. Western blot showing induction of CYP1A1 protein in IGROV-1 xenograft tumors retrieved from mice treated with Phortress (20 mg/kg; 24 h). Tumor lysates were prepared and proteins separated by PAGE: Lane 1, +ve control, 5 μg CYP1A1 microsomes; lanes 2 and 3, untreated and vehicle control-treated samples; lanes 4 and 5, 24 h 20 mg/kg Phortress [36].

in transcriptional activation of target genes including CYP1A1 and CYP1B1 in breast cancer cells sensitive to this agent [28]. As 5F 203 causes IGROV-1 cytotoxicity and consistent with the hypothesis that 5F 203 is an AhR agonist ligand [47], we wished to determine whether 5F 203 activates AhR signaling in IGROV-1 cells with resulting AhR translocation from cytoplasm to nucleus.

The effect of 5F 203 (1 μM) on subcellular distribution of immunoreactive AhR protein was studied by Western blot. We demonstrated (**Figure 4A**), in IGROV-1 cells treated with DMSO only, the cytoplasmic fraction contained relatively high levels of AhR protein compared with the nuclear fraction. In contrast, after treatment of cells with AhR agonists, 1 μM 5F 203 or 10 nM TCDD (positive control), between 1 and 6 h, immunoreactive AhR protein could be detected in the nuclear fraction, indicating AhR translocation [48].

To identify whether 5F 203 caused AhR nuclear translocation in 5F 203-insensitive ovarian carcinoma cells, the effect of 5F 203 (1 μM) on subcellular distribution of immunoreactive AhR protein was assessed by Western blot in SKOV-3 cells. In DMSO-treated cells, AhR protein levels were high in cytoplasmic and nuclear fractions. After treatment with 1 μM 5F 203 (0.5–6 h), AhR protein in SKOV-3 cytoplasm remained unchanged. AhR was already present in SKOV-3 nuclei and further translocation was negligible.

After treatment with TCDD, although cytoplasmic AhR was lost, there was no evidence of AhR gain in nuclear fractions (**Figure 4A**). These results were confirmed by immunofluorescence of AhR.

It was then logical to investigate putative activation of CYP1A1-related promoter sequences in 5F 203-sensitive ovarian cancer cells.

CYP1A1 and CYP1B1 promoters are regulated by AhR, which forms a heterodimer with the AhR nuclear transporter (ARNT). Binding of the complete dimer to XRE promoter regions mediates transcription of AhR-responsive genes, including CYP1A1. IGROV-1 and SKOV-3 were transfected with XRE-luciferase reporter construct (pTX.Dir), as a control, the same reporter construct without XRE elements (pT81) was used. Cells were then treated with 0.1% DMSO, 0.1–1 μM 5F 203 or TCDD 10 nM. In IGROV-1 cells transfected with pTX.Dir, 5.5-fold induction of luciferase activity was observed when cells were treated with 1 μM 5F 203 (**Figure 4B**).

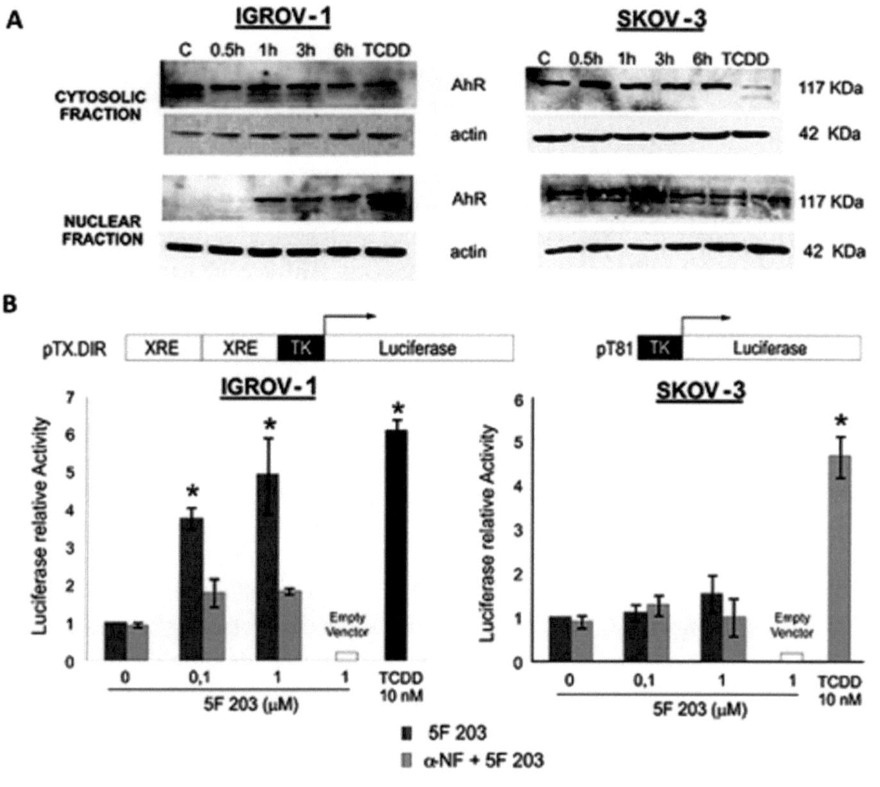

Figure 4.
5F 203 induces AhR nuclear translocation and activation of CYP1A1-related promoter sequences in sensitive ovarian cancer cell lines. A: AhR Subcellular localization. IGROV-1 and SKOV-3 cells were incubated with 5F 203 (1 μM) for indicated times, DMSO (0.1%) for 6 h or TCDD (10 nM) for 1 h as a positive control. Nuclear and cytosolic fractions were isolated using a commercial kit and analyzed for AhR content by Western blot. The figure shows representative Western blots. All Western blots were performed three times for each cell line and revealed the same pattern of AhR subcellular distribution. B: Activation of CYP1A1-related promoter sequences. Cells were transfected with a plasmid containing XRE (AhR consensus sequences) upstream of the luciferase reporter gene and a second plasmid containing R. reniformis luciferase gene as an internal control. After 24 h, cells were incubated with 5F 203 for 18 h or pre-treated for 1 h with 1 μM α-NF followed by 18 h of 5F 203 plus 1 μM α-NF. Luciferase activity was determined using the Dual-Luciferase Reporter Assay System (Promega). Values represent the average of three independent experiments.

No induction in luciferase activity was observed when SKOV-3 cells transfected with pTX.Dir were treated with 5F 203 (1 μM). Cells transfected with pT81 and treated with 1 μM 5F 203 showed negligible luciferase activity induction (1.1-fold).

These findings clearly demonstrated that 5F 203 induces activation of promoter sequences known to respond to AhR-mediated signals. This is consistent with interaction of protein complexes induced by treatment with 5F 203 through the XRE CYP1A1 promoter sequence.

In IGROV-1 cells, pre-treatment (1 h) with AhR antagonist α-NF (1 μM) followed by co-treatment (18 h) with 5F 203 plus 1 μM α-NF reduced induction (2.65-fold) of luciferase activity. These results support the requirement of AhR in increased XRE-luciferase activity [48].

1.6 5F 203-induced ROS and γH2AX foci formation in sensitive cells is mediated by AhR

Previous studies demonstrated CYP1A1 induction by 5F 203, and CYP catalyzed 5F 203 biotransformation to DNA reactive species [40]. CYP activity contributed to increased intracellular ROS levels [49]. Oxidative stress is involved in various biological processes including proliferation and apoptosis. Therefore, we compared the effect of 5F 203 on ROS production in Bz-sensitive IGROV-1 cells and Bz-insensitive SKOV-3 cells. To determine whether 5F 203 altered intracellular ROS levels, cells were treated with 5F 203 for 6 h and exposed to 2,7-DCF before ROS levels were evaluated using flow cytometry. 5F 203 increased ROS levels in IGROV-1 cells only. This effect, detectable following 1 h of 1 μM 5F 203 treatment, was partially blocked by pre-incubation of cells with α-NF (**Figure 5A**). Also, pre-treatment with ROS inhibitors N-acetyl cysteine (NAC) and Trolox partially decreased the effect of 5F 203 in IGROV-1 cells (**Figure 5B**). In contrast, 5F 203 strongly inhibited ROS production in SKOV-3 cells, despite detection of neither phenotypic changes nor AhR translocation [48].

It is reported that ROS may cause activation of nuclear factor kappa B (NF-κB) [50]. As activation of this pathway induces NF-κB nuclear translocation, we performed immunostaining of NF-κB using a specific antibody in IGROV-1 and SKOV-3 cells before and after treatment with 5F 203. 5F 203 induced NF-κB translocation in IGROV-1 cells only, and this effect was prevented by pre-treatment of cells with 1 μM α-NF. We then investigated whether 5F 203 caused DNA damage. To determine DNA double-strand breaks (DSB), γH2AX foci were measured in IGROV-1 and SKOV-3 cells following exposure to 5F 203 (1 μM, 2–4 h). DNA DSB formation precipitates serine 139 phosphorylation of histone H2AX, producing γH2AX at DSB sites [48]. γH2AX foci appeared within nuclei of IGROV-1 cells only following treatment with 5F 203 (1 μM; 2–4 h; **Figure 5C**). Foci formation was partially blocked by pre-treatment of cells with α-NF, confirming that activation of AhR is needed for 5F 203-induced DNA damage. In contrast, neither vehicle-treated cells nor SKOV-3 cells challenged with 5F 203 displayed γH2AX foci within their nuclei at any time point examined. These data are consistent with neutral COMET assays performed to examine DNA damage (double-strand breaks) wrought as a consequence of dose-dependent DNA adduct generation which has been detected following treatment of IGROV-1 cells *in vitro* with 5F 203 or Phortress, and in IGROV-1 xenografts retrieved from tumor-bearing mice exposed to Phortress [36].

1.7 5F 203 modulates expression and phosphorylation of stress MAPKs

Mitogen-activated protein kinases (MAPKs) can be modulated by many factors including cell lesions induced by DNA damage [51]. We therefore investigated the effect of 5F 203 on activation of these protein kinases in IGROV-1 cells. As depicted

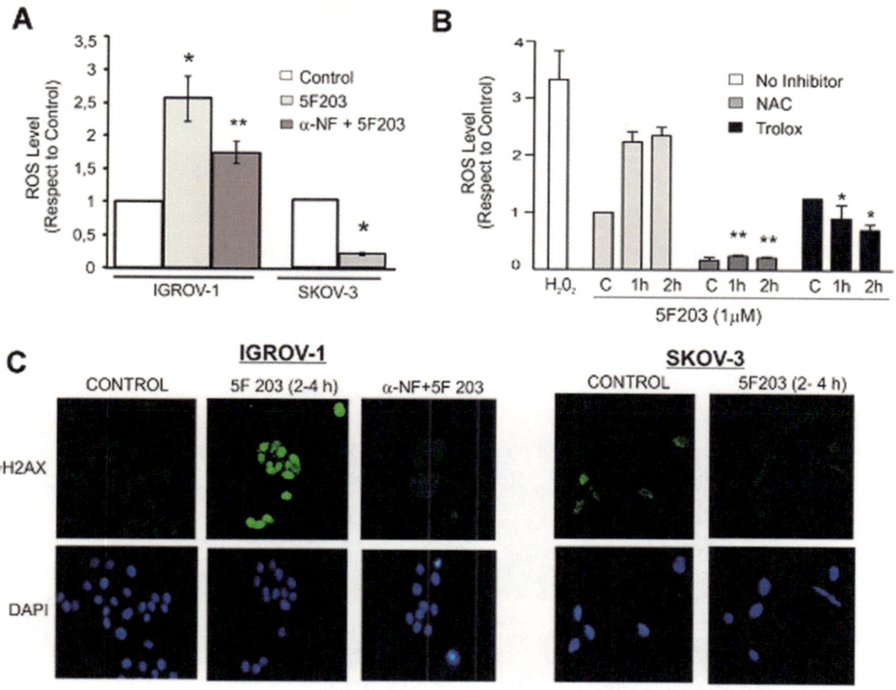

Figure 5.
*5F 203 increases ROS levels. Exponentially growing IGROV-1 and SKOV-3 cells were treated with 5F 203 (1 μM) or vehicle control (0.1% DMSO) continuously for 1, 2, 4, or 6 h and ROS levels were measured by flow cytometry after incubation with 2,7-DCF. Data represent the mean of at least two independent experiments where n = 2 per experiment; bars, SEM. *P < 0.05 when compared to untreated cells, **P < 0.05 when compared to cells treated without AhR inhibitor. B: Trolox and NAC inhibition of 5F 203-mediated ROS induction. IGROV-1 cells were exposed to 0.1% DMSO (control), 5F 203 (1 μM) for 1 or 2 h, or pre-treated with Trolox (250 μM) or NAC (100 μM) for 1 h followed by 5F 203 (1 μM) inhibitor for 1 or 2 h. ROS levels were measured by fluorometry after incubation with 2,7-DCF. Data represent the mean of at least two independent experiments where n = 2 per experiment; bars, SEM. *P < 0.05 or **P < 0.01 when compared to cells treated without ROS inhibitor. C: Induces γH2AX foci formation in sensitive IGROV-1 cells. A: Measurement of ROS levels. γH2AX foci following 2–4 h of treatment of cells with 5F 203 (1 μM); IGROV-1 cell nuclei were stained with DAPI. Stained cells were visualized on a fluorescence Nikon C1 confocal microscope using a 60X PlanApo AN 0.95 objective, images were processed and analyzed with Nikon C1-EZ package, version 2.20.*

in **Figure 6A**, 5F 203 induced phosphorylation of JNK and P38, the stronger effect was attained after 6 h of treatment in both cases. Also, treatment with 5F 203 increased P38 α levels. Pre-treatment of cells with α-NF decreased phosphorylation of these kinases and P38 α expression, which confirmed that 5F 203 affected expression and activation of these proteins through AhR activation. Exposure to 5F 203 (1 h) also increased phosphorylation of ERK in IGROV-1 cells.

The ability of 5F 203 to induce apoptosis was evaluated. Exposure of IGROV-1 cells to 5F 203 (1 μM; 24 h) induced apoptotic body formation (**Figure 6B**). In contrast, SKOV-3 cells, resistant to 5F 203, did not show such features (**Figure 6B**). Also, pre-treatment of cells with α-NF partially blocked the pro-apoptotic effect of 5F 203 in IGROV-1 cells. These data confirmed that AhR is involved in 5F 203-induced cell death [48].

Trolox (a vitamin E derivative) and NAC are potent ROS scavengers often used as antioxidant agents. We pre-treated IGROV-1 cells with Trolox or NAC in order to investigate the effect of ROS depletion on 5F 203-induced growth inhibition. Cells were exposed to 5F 203 (1 μM, 24 h) after pre-treatment with Trolox (250 μM) or NAC (100 μM) for 1 h. As observed in **Figure 6B,** both inhibitors partially reduced 5F 203-induced apoptotic body formation. These data support the involvement of ROS-generation in 5F 203-induced apoptosis in sensitive IGROV-1 cells [48].

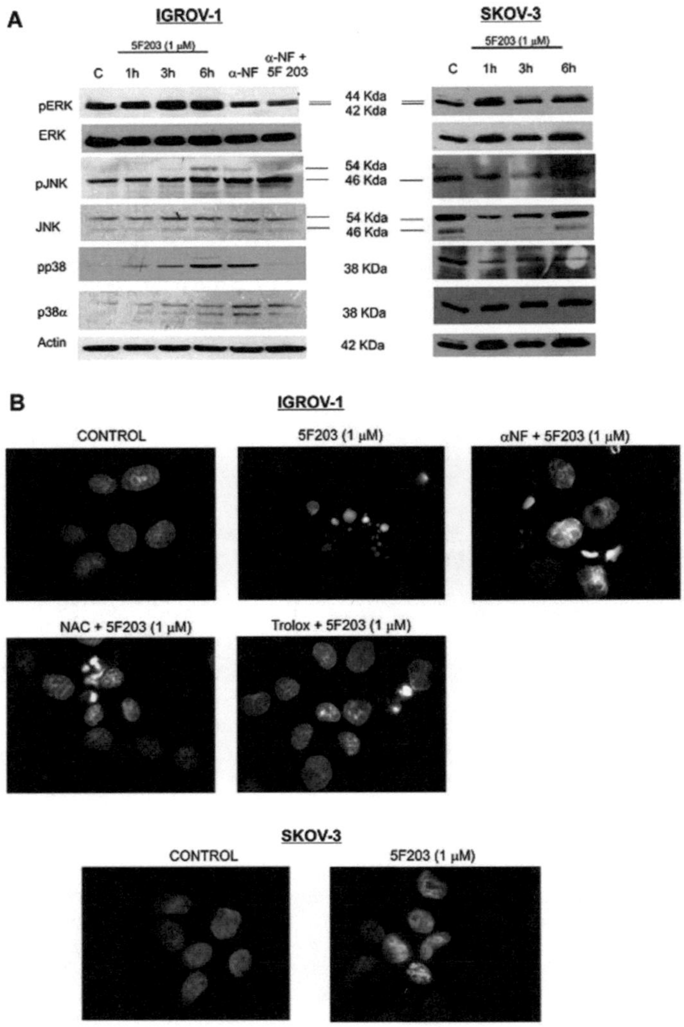

Figure 6.
5F 203 induces MAPK activation and apoptosis in sensitive IGROV-1 cells. A: MAPK expression and activation. IGROV-1 and SKOV-3 cells were incubated with 5F203 (1 μM) for indicated times or DMSO (0.1%) for 6 h. Whole cell extracts were obtained and subjected to SDS-PAGE and Western blotting with pERK, ERK, pJNK, JNK, pp38, and p38 α antibodies. The figure shows representative Western blots. All Western blots were performed three times for each cell line and revealed the same pattern of protein phosphorylation and expression. B: Evaluation of cell apoptosis. Cells were incubated with 1 μM 5F 203 or DMSO (0.1%) for 24 h or pre-treated with α-NF (1 μM) Trolox (250 μM) or NAC (100 μM) for 1 h followed by 5F 203 (1 μM) for 24 h. Then, non-adherent cells were obtained by cytocentrifugation in the culture medium. Once fixed, cells were stained with DAPI and observed under a fluorescence microscope. Condensed and fragmented nuclei were considered apoptotic. Representative fields are shown.

1.8 5F 203 alters cell cycle distribution and evokes apoptosis in sensitive ovarian cancer cells

As results indicated that 5F 203 induced DNA damage (e.g., **Figure 6B**), perturbations in cell cycle were explored. IGROV-1 and SKOV-3 cells were exposed to 1 μM 5F 203 or 0.1% DMSO for 24 and 48 h and prepared for cell cycle analyses. As illustrated (**Figure 7A**), 5F 203 caused an increase in G1 phase IGROV-1 events (44% control; 50% at 24 h and 59% at 48 h), coinciding with decreased G2/M phase (20% control to 13% at 24 h and 9% at 48 h). Accumulation of sub-G1 events was also detected from 5% (control) to 12 and 20% at 24 and 48 h, respectively. When cells were pre-incubated with α-NF, sub-G1 events diminished, indicating that AhR

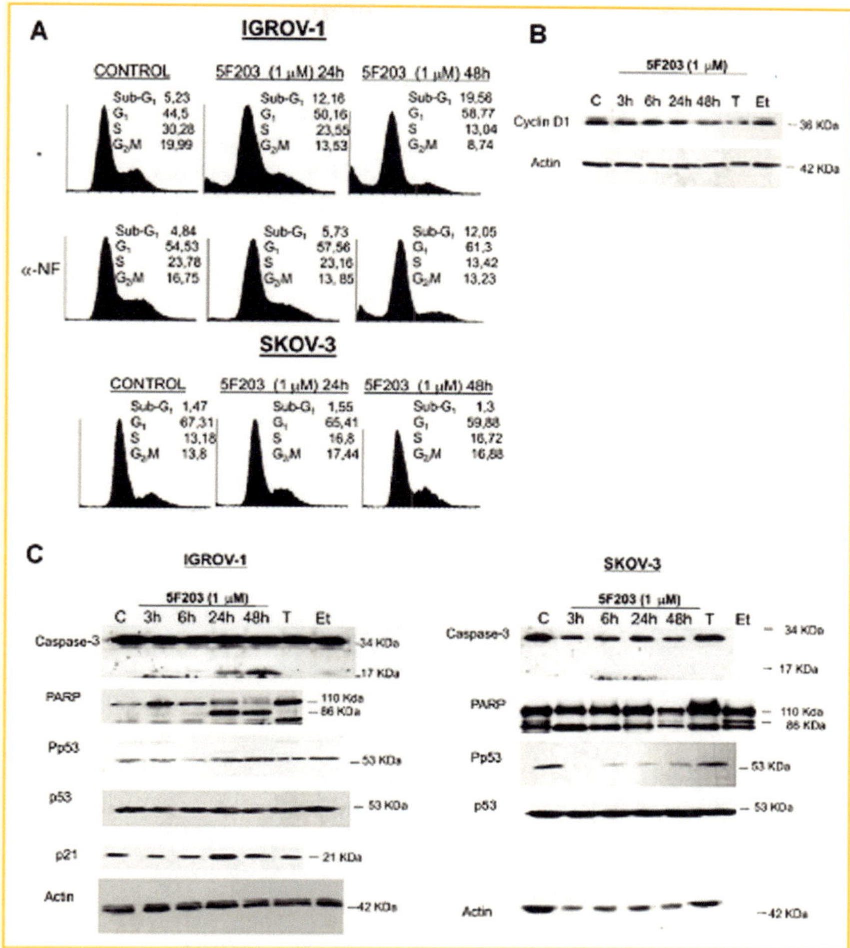

Figure 7.
5F 203 induces AhR-dependent cell cycle arrest in G1 phase, a decrease in cyclin D1 and caspase-3 mediated apoptosis in sensitive ovarian cancer cells. A: Exponentially growing IGROV-1 cells were exposed to either 0.1% DMSO (control) or 5F 203 (1 μM) for 24 and 48 h, (upper panel) or pre-incubated for 1 h with -α NF followed by 24 or 48 h 5F 203 +α -NF (1 μM) (lower panel). Exponentially growing SKOV-3 cells were exposed to either 0.1% DMSO (control) or 5F203 (1 μM) for 24 or 48 h. Then both cell lines were harvested, washed in PBS, and fixed in 70% ethanol. DNA was stained by incubating cells in PBS containing propidium iodide and fluorescence measured and analyzed as described in Materials and Methods section. The experiment was repeated three times (significant difference between treatments with p <0.01). Data of one representative experiment are shown in the figure. B: Effect of 5F 203 on cyclin D1 expression. IGROV-1 cells were exposed to either 0.1% DMSO (control) or 5F 203 (1 μM) for 3, 6, 24, or 48 h. Proteins in total lysates were resolved by SDS-PAGE and Western blot performed with anti-cyclin D1 Ab. Anti-actin Ab was used as a loading control. C: Effect of 5F 203 on p53 signaling pathway, caspase-3 activation, and PARP cleavage in ovarian cancer cells. Cells were incubated with 1 μM 5F 203 during indicated times or TCDD (T) 10 nM for 1 h. Cells treated with 10 μM Etoposide (Et) were used as a positive control for apoptosis. Whole cell extracts were obtained and subjected to SDS-PAGE and Western blotting with pp53 and P21, caspase-3 and PARP antibodies. PP53, phosphorylated form of P53.

activation is necessary for 5F 203-induced apoptosis. In contrast, SKOV-3 cell cycle was not perturbed following treatment with 5F 203.The data demonstrate that 5F 203-induced DNA damage may lead to accumulation of cells in G1 phase concomitant with growth inhibition. As IGROV-1 cells are p53 wild type, their response to 5F 203 is consistent with operation of a G1 checkpoint arrest to cell cycle progression after DNA damage. As G1 phase arrest was observed in 5F 203-sensitive cells, cyclin D1 levels were examined. Exposure of IGROV-1 cells to 5F 203 reduced cyclin D1 protein levels by 50 and 75% after 24 and 48 h, respectively. In contrast, only a 35% decrease in cyclin D1 levels was observed in SKOV-3 cells after 48 h treatment with

5F 203 (**Figure 7B**). In order to study, whether 5F 203 treatment caused caspase 3 activation, PARP cleavage, and p53 phosphorylation in IGROV-1 cells as a result of its pro-apoptotic action, we carried out Western blot experiments upon separated proteins of whole cell lysates following treatment of cells with 1 μM 5F 203 between 3 and 48 h. We observed caspase-3 activation, PARP cleavage, and 2.7- and 4-fold increase in p53 phosphorylation between 24 and 48 h, respectively. A similar pattern of increased p21 protein levels was observed after treatment of IGROV-1 cells

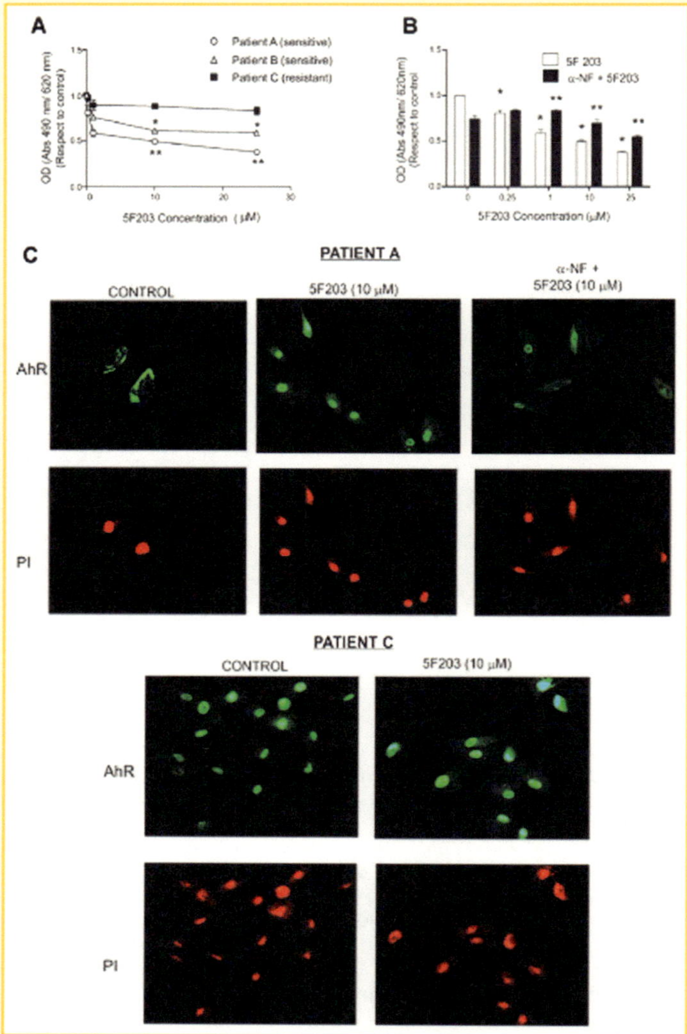

Figure 8.
*5F 203 activity in ascites-derived ovarian cancer cell strains isolated from patients. A: 5F 203 cytotoxicity assay. Cells derived from three patients were incubated with 5F 203 for 5 days. Cellular viability was evaluated by MTS assay. Values represent the average of two independent experiments using cells from one patient with n = 4, *P < 0.05 compared with untreated cells. B: Cells derived from patient A (sensitive to 5F 203) were incubated with 5F 203 for 5 days or pre-treated for 1 h with α-NF (1 μM) and then treated with 5F 203 plus α-NF (1 μM) for 5 days. Cellular viability was evaluated by MTS assay. The values represent the average of two independent experiments using cells from one patient with n = 4, **P < 0.01 compared with cells incubated without AhR inhibitor. C: 5F 203 induces translocation of AhR to the nucleus in sensitive ascites-derived ovarian cancer cells. The staining of cells from one representative patient is shown. Cells were grown on coverslips and treated with DMSO for 1 h, 5F 203 for 30 min, or α-NF (1 μM) followed by 1 h of 5F 203, α-NF (1 μM), or 10 nM TCDD for 1 h. After fixation, cells were double-stained for AhR (green) and propidium iodide (red). Cells treated with 10 nM TCDD were incubated only with secondary antibody to determine non-specific background. Stained cells were visualized on a fluorescence microscope using a 40X PlanApo AN 0.95 objective, and images were processed and analyzed with Nikon C1-EZ package, version 2.20.*

with 5F 203 (**Figure 7C**). In contrast, caspase activation and PARP cleavage were not detected in SKOV-3 cells treated with 5F 203; these cells showed decreased levels of pp53 after treatment with 5F 203 (**Figure 7C**) [48].

Thus, clear distinction can be seen—in terms of AhR signal transduction activation, CYP1A1 induction, DNA damage, ROS generation and apoptosis—between Bz-sensitive and Bz-insensitive ovarian cancer models *in vitro* and *in vivo*. It is important to evaluate whether such distinction can be translated to the clinic to enable identification of sensitive ovarian cancer phenotypes.

1.9 5F 203-induced cytotoxicity in cells isolated from ovarian cancer ascites is mediated by AhR

It has been proposed that high-grade advanced stage papillary serous ovarian adenocarcinoma ascites fluid is enriched for "metastatic," or "tumor-initiating" cells, and that these cells may represent a therapy-resistant population. Thus, ascites is considered a good model for disease study [52]. Cancer cells derived from ascites fluid produced by ovarian tumors from three patients were authenticated by pathologists. All tumors were high-grade (G3), serous, papillary histological type. Cells were treated *ex vivo* with 5F 203 for 5 days and cytotoxicity measured using MTS assays. Two cell strains were sensitive to 5F 203 and one was resistant (**Figure 8A**). In patient A, 1 and 10 μM 5F 203 decreased cell viability by 40 and 50%, respectively (compared to control considered 100%). This decrease in cell viability diminished to 20 and 30%, respectively, when cells were pre-treated with 1 μM α-NF followed by incubation with 5F 203/α-NF. We observed similar results in cells derived from patient B (data not shown). Results indicate that AhR mediates the effect of 5F 203 in these papillary tumors sensitive to 5F 203 (**Figure 8B**). AhR localization and nuclear translocation were then investigated. As demonstrated in **Figure 4A**, in ovarian cancer cells treated with vehicle (DMSO), high levels of cytosolic AhR protein were detected with some nuclear AhR staining present. However, after treatment for just 1 h with 1 μM 5F 203 or 10 nM TCDD, immunofluorescent AhR protein levels increased in the nucleus and decreased in the cytosol. In contrast, constitutive nuclear AhR localization was detected in cells of patient C, resistant to 5F 203. CYP1A1 mRNA levels were measured by real-time PCR in cells from patients A, B (sensitive to 5F 203), and C (resistant to 5F 203) following exposure to 5F 203 (1 μM; 24 h). In cells from patients A and B, we observed induction of *cyp1a1* expression (**Figure 8A**), which was partially reduced by α-NF. In contrast, reduction of (constitutive) *cyp1a1* expression was observed after treatment of patient C cells with 5F 203. ROS levels were also evaluated after treatment of patient ascites cells with 5F 203 and increased levels were detected only in cells sensitive to 5F 203, ROS were not induced in the 5F 203-insensitive ascites cells of patient C (**Figure 8B**) [48].

These promising data represent only a small clinical sample, but nevertheless support the hypothesis that in a clinical setting, "patient selection" and "precision medicine" are models applicable to antitumor Bzs.

2. Discussion

In this chapter, we propose that AhR represents a novel molecular target for ovarian cancer treatment and that the Bz class signifies AhR-targeted, CYP-activated anticancer agents for the treatment of ovarian cancer.

5F 203 activates AhR signaling in cultured and patient ovarian carcinoma cells sensitive to this agent, demonstrating that 5F 203 cytotoxicity is AhR dependent. In sensitive IGROV-1 cells, 5F 203, a known AhR ligand [35], triggers

AhR translocation from cytosol to nucleus, activating CYP1A1-related promoter sequences driving transcription of AhR-responsive genes as reported by XRE-luciferase.

It was recognized several years ago that certain ovarian cancer cell lines were exquisitely sensitive to antitumor Bzs [32]. 5F 203 potency and selectivity against ovarian cell lines within the NCI panel have been demonstrated [32, 53]: IGROV-1, OVCAR4 and OVCAR5 displayed GI_{50} values <100 nM in contrast, whereas GI_{50} values >100 μM were observed in OVCAR8 and SKOV-3 cell lines. Subsequently, induction of CYP1A1 by 5F 203 in sensitive cancer cells only inferred significant correlation between sensitivity and CYP1A1 induction [48]. *In vivo*, significant antitumor efficacy of 5F 203 prodrug Phortress was demonstrated against IGROV-1 ovarian (as well as breast) tumor xenografts. Moreover, CYP1A1 expression was detected in IGROV-1 (and sensitive breast) tumors of mice receiving Phortress treatment. No CYP1A1 protein was detected in insensitive breast tumor tissue following treatment of mice with Phortress [36]. Phortress was well tolerated, it possessed excellent solubility, bioavailability, and pharmacokinetic properties (liberating efficacious, sustained 5F 203 plasma concentrations), and Phase 1 clinical trials were initiated. Clinical evaluation revealed long-term stable disease in lung, colorectal, and kidney cancer patients; however, neither ovarian nor breast cancer patients were recruited to trial and short patent life precluded continuation of development.

AhR ligands such as 5F 203 induce their own CYP-catalyzed bioactivation; therefore, potential drug-drug or indeed drug-xenobiotic interactions were considered prior to commencement of the clinical trial. For example, many oral contraceptives are steroid based and any drug inducing CYP1A1 activity will lead to rapid metabolism and reduced contraceptive efficacy [54]. In the Phortress trial protocol, it was cautioned not to drink grapefruit juice, as this is able to inhibit CYP1A1 potentially reducing Phortress efficacy [55]. Red wine consumption was also discouraged as resveratrol is a competitive antagonist of AhR ligands; it promotes AhR nuclear translocation and binding to DNA, but transactivation of AhR-inducible genes such as *cyp1a1* is inhibited [56].

Differential sensitivity to 5F 203 may be a consequence of differential regulation by AhR of CYP1A1 expression in different cell types. In resistant cells, we observed constitutive nuclear localization of AhR. In resistant cells, AhR may be associated with co-repressors [57]; lack of AhR degradation (by ubiquitination) or recycling may lead to inappropriate AhR function [58]. Also, different AhR nuclear localization sequences [57] or polymorphisms may cause inappropriate receptor function [59]. Additionally, mutations in the CYP1A1 promoter in insensitive cells may lead to decreased CYP1A1 activation [60, 61]. Considering the clinical potential of 5F 203, its mechanism of action was further investigated. 5F 203 induced ROS formation in sensitive cells (**Figure 5**). In IGROV-1 cells, 5F 203 evoked DNA damage detected as H2AX foci (2–4 h), increased pp53 levels and P21 expression, decreased cyclin D1 expression, caused G1 cell cycle arrest and apoptosis. In contrast, SKOV-3 cells showed decreased levels of pp53 after treatment with 5F 203; the reason for this effect is unclear, but it may contribute to cellular resistance to 5F 203 (**Figure 7**). 5F 203-induced growth inhibition and apoptosis in IGROV-1 cells may in part be a consequence of elevated ROS (**Figure 5A**) and caspase-3 activation (**Figure 7C**) resulting in oxidative DNA damage and cell death [48]. Oxidative stress may activate caspases and is implicated in a number of cellular processes including apoptosis. Many chemotherapeutic agents are known to induce cytotoxicity by ROS-mediated mechanisms, for example, doxorubicin [62] and AhR ligand aminoflavone [63]. It was demonstrated that ROS might trigger apoptosis signaling mediated by p53 in IGROV-1 cells [64–66]. IGROV-1 cells possess wild type p53 and show sensitivity

to 5F 203. However, 5F 203 activity is independent of p53 exemplified by (i) potent activity of 5F 203 in MDA-MB-468 p53 mutant cells [32] and (ii) IGROV-1 variant populations demonstrating acquired resistance to cisplatin retaining sensitivity to 5F 203 (Bradshaw et al. unpublished results). Cisplatin resistance is associated with p53 mutations in IGROV-1 cells [64]. In IGROV-1 cells, p53 may be attempting (failed) repair rather than mediating apoptosis. Our results show that antioxidant agents such as NAC and Trolox decrease ROS formation and protect IGROV-1 cells from apoptosis induced by 5F 203 (**Figure 5B**). Previous work has demonstrated that stress signaling pathways are also activated by cisplatin and retinoids in IGROV-1 and cisplatin-resistant IGROV-1 cells; furthermore activation of JNK and P38 by these agents is stronger in cisplatin-resistant IGROV-1 cells. Reflecting the integral to antitumor activity, 5F 203 induces ROS in sensitive IGROV-1 cells and that IGROV-1 cells resistant to cisplatin retain sensitivity to 5F 203, we propose that 5F 203 could be a putative treatment for ovarian tumors. MAPK p38 α acts as an oxidative stress sensor; ROS-induced activation of p38 promotes apoptosis and prevents further oncogenic/carcinogenic ROS formation [44]. Also, micro-RNAs (miRNA) expression can be altered by different stress conditions, and they are well-known stress response regulators. It has been described that two members of the miR-200 family, miR-141 and miR-200a, inhibit p38 α and have an essential role in the redox response. In animal models, accumulation of miRNAs mimics p38 α deficiency and promotes malignancy. Human ovarian adenocarcinomas demonstrating high oxidative stress show high expression of miR-200a and low basal levels of p38 α. Chemotherapy drugs that induce ROS also induce p38 α in these tumors, leading to apoptosis. It was proposed that in ovarian tumors, high levels of miR-200 s and low levels of p38 α could be predictive markers of good clinical response to chemotherapy [45]. Our results are consistent with these observations, IGROV-1 cells have low levels of basal p38 α and treatment with 5F 203 induced p38 α expression and pp38 (**Figure 6A**), which may lead to apoptosis. In contrast, SKOV-3 cells show high basal levels of p38 α and treatment with 5F 203 did not modulate p38 α expression or activation (**Figure 6A**).
We hypothesize that this may contribute to the lack of apoptosis induction in SKOV-3 cells. Finally, compatible with results from ovarian cancer cell lines, we identified putative surrogate markers of sensitivity to 5F 203 in a small sample of patient tumors. Clear distinction was demonstrated between ovarian cancer patient tumor cells that were sensitive to 5F 203 and those that were inherently 5F 203-resistant. Only in ascites-isolated patient tumor cells sensitive to 5F 203 were (i) cytosolic AhR translocation to cell nuclei, (ii) CYP1A1 mRNA induction, and (iii) increased ROS levels observed (**Figures 8** and **9**) in response to *ex vivo* treatment. Such pharmacodynamic endpoints are readily obtained from bioassays that could be adopted clinically to detect candidate 5F 203-responsive patients. In this way, unresponsive patients would be spared unnecessary treatment. Sensitivity to 5F 203 and AhR activation should be examined in a larger sample of ovarian carcinoma patient tumors of different histological types in future studies (**Figure 10**). However, the fact that cells isolated from patients with high-grade ovarian tumors were sensitive to 5F 203 shows that this agent may offer alternative treatment for patients with advanced disease. Intraperitoneal (i.p.) chemotherapy is currently used in treatment of ovarian tumors, and both 5F 203 and its prodrug Phortress have demonstrated antitumor efficacy administered either intravenously or i.p. [34].

Nanoformulations of 5F 203 are currently under evaluation to maximize tumor-targeting and sustained, controlled release. Future studies will include investigation of miRNA profiles in 5F 203-sensitive ovarian cancer cells compared with those of insensitive ones. In addition, the activity of 5F 203 against ovarian cancer stem cell-like/initiating populations remains to be evaluated.

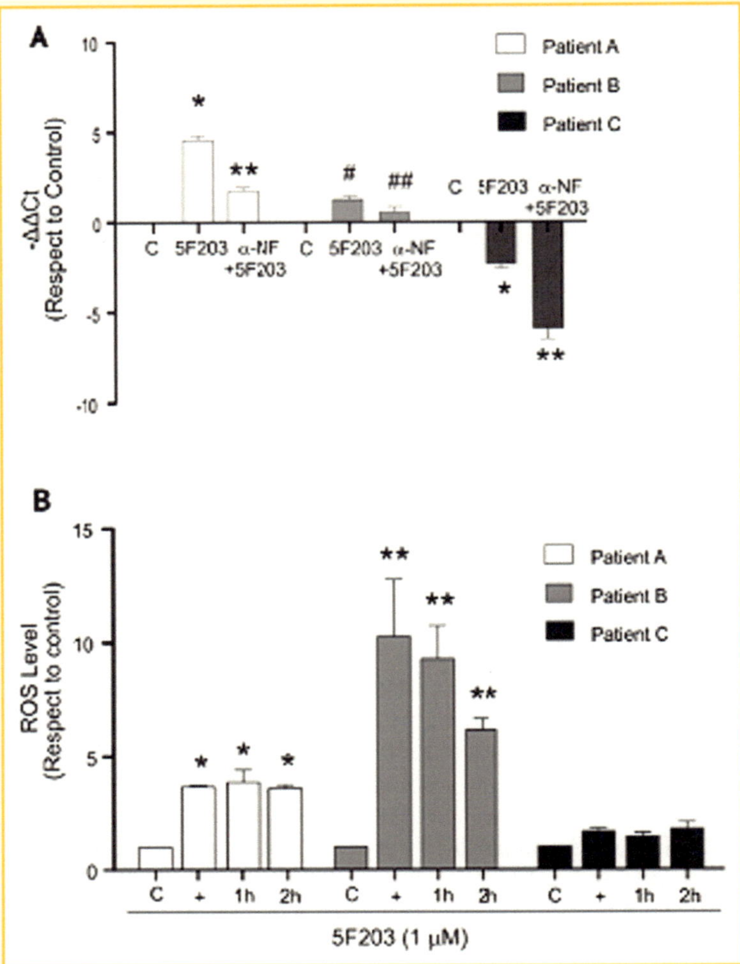

Figure 9.
*5F 203 induces CYP1A1 over-expression and increases ROS levels in sensitive ascites-derived ovarian cancer cells isolated from patients. A: Induction of CYP1A1 gene expression. Cells derived from three patients were exposed to 0.1% DMSO (control), 5F 203 (1 μM) for 24 h, or pre-treated with α-NF (1 μM) for 1 h followed by 5F 203 (1 μM) α-NF (1 μM) for 24 h. RNA was isolated and real-time PCR was performed to measure CYP1A1 expression. A: Each bar represents mean ± SD of triplicate measurements in drug treated, compared to untreated cells, using GAPDH expression as an endogenous control. *P < 0.01 or *P < 0.05 when compared to untreated cells **P < 0.01 or **P < 0.05 when compared to cells treated without AhR inhibitor. B: Measurement of ROS levels. Cells derived from three patients were treated with 5F 203 (1 μM) or vehicle control (0.1% DMSO) continuously for 1 or 2 h and ROS levels were measured by fluorometry after incubation with 2,7-DCF. Incubation with H2O2 (100 μM) was used as positive control. Data represent the mean of at least two independent experiments where n = 4 per experiment; bars, SEM. *P < 0.05, **P < 0.01 when compared to untreated cells.*

In summary, we have demonstrated AhR-dependent cytotoxicity of 5F 203 in ovarian carcinoma cells, we conclude that AhR may represent a new molecular target in the treatment of ovarian cancer and that 5F 203 may offer a potential novel treatment for newly diagnosed and cisplatin-resistant disease.

Tumor cells will be isolated from ascites fluid and cultured *ex vivo*. Following exposure of carcinoma cells *ex vivo* to escalating Bz concentrations (i) Bz sensitivity; (ii) AhR localization and nuclear translocation; (iii) CYP 1A1 expression and inducibility (by Bz); and (iv) ROS generation will be determined. If tumor cells are identified that show dose-dependent growth inhibition, AhR translocation,

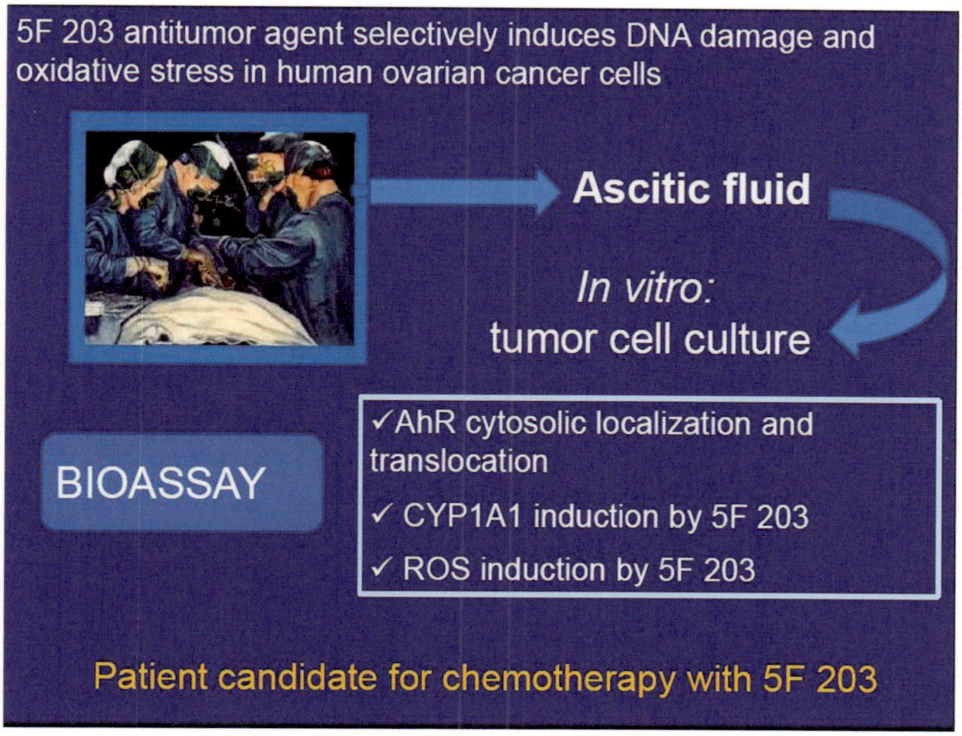

Figure 10.
Proposed procedure for identification of patients whose tumors may be responsive to Bz treatment.

CYP 1A1 induction, and ROS generation following exposure to Bz, the patient from whom cells were isolated may be identified as a suitable candidate to receive Bz therapy.

Acknowledgements

We are very grateful to Dr. Eduardo Sandes from Área de Investigaciones, Instituto de Oncología "Ángel H. Roffo," Universidad de Buenos Aires, for his assistance with figures.

Author details

Andrea I. Loaiza Perez[1,2]* and Tracey D. Bradshaw[3]

1 National Scientific Council (CONICET), Ciudad de Buenos Aires, Argentina

2 Área de Investigaciones, Instituto de Oncología "Ángel H. Roffo", Universidad de Buenos Aires, Ciudad de Buenos Aires, Argentina

3 Centre for Biomolecular Science, University of Nottingham, Nottingham, UK

*Address all correspondence to: loaizaa2012@gmail.com

References

[1] https://www.cancer.gov/types/ovarian

[2] https://www.wcrf.org/dietandcancer/cancers

[3] Bast RC Jr, Hennessy B, Mills GB. The biology of ovarian cancer: New opportunities for translation. Nature Reviews. Cancer. 2009;**9**:415-428

[4] Hennessy BT, Murph M, Nanjundan M, Carey M, Auersperg N, Almeida J, et al. Ovarian cancer: Linking genomics to new target discovery and molecular markers--the way ahead. Advances in Experimental Medicine and Biology. 2008;**617**:23-40

[5] Colombo N, Lorusso D, Scollo P. Impact of recurrence of ovarian cancer on quality of life and outlook for the future. International Journal of Cancer. 2017;**27**(6):1134-1140

[6] Gorringe KL, Campbell IG. Large-scale genomic analysis of ovarian carcinomas. Molecular Oncology. 2009;**3**:157-164

[7] Gray JW, Suzuki S, Kuo WL, Polikoff D, Deavers M, Smith-McCune K, et al. Specific keynote: Genome copynumber abnormalities in ovarian cancer. Gynecologic Oncology. 2003;**88**:S16-S21; Discussion S22-14

[8] Nanjundan M, Cheng KW, Zhang F, Lahad J, Kuo WL, Schmandt R, et al. Overexpression of SnoN/SkiL, amplified at the 3q26.2 locus, in ovarian cancers: A role in ovarian pathogenesis. Molecular Oncology. 2008;**2**:164-181

[9] Rossi L, Verrico M, Zaccarelli E, Papa A, Colonna M, Strudel M, et al. Bevacizumab in ovarian cancer: A critical review of phase III studies. Oncotarget. 2017;**8**(7):12389-12405. DOI: 10.18632/oncotarget.13310

[10] Kehoe S. Olaparib and ovarian cancer—Overall survival outcomes. The Lancet Oncology. 1 Nov 2016;**17**(11):1474-1475. DOI: 10.1016/S1470-2045(16)30433-8

[11] https://www.cancer.gov/news-events/cancer-currents-blog/2017/fda-niraparib-ovarian

[12] Nebert DW. Aryl hydrocarbon receptor (AHR): "pioneer member" of the basic-helix/loop/helix per-Arnt-sim (bHLH/PAS) family of "sensors" of foreign and endogenous signals. Progress in Lipid Research. 2017;**67**:38-57. DOI: 10.1016/j.plipres.2017.06.001. Epub 2017 Jun 9

[13] McGuire J, Coumailleau P, Whitelaw ML, et al. The basic helix-loop-helix/PAS factor Sim is associated with hsp90: Implications for regulation by interaction with partner factors. Journal of Biological Chemistry. 1995;**270**(52):31353-31357

[14] Fukunaga BN, Probst MR, Reisz-Porszasz S, Hankinson O. Identification of functional domains of the aryl hydrocarbon receptor. Journal of Biological Chemistry. 1995;**270**(49):29270-29278

[15] Antonsson C, Whitelaw ML, McGuire J, et al. Distinct roles of the molecular chaperone hsp90 in modulating dioxin receptor function via the basic helix-loop-helix and PAS domains. Molecular and Cellular Biology. 1995;**15**(2):756-765

[16] Wang GL, Jiang BH, Rue EA, Semenza GL. Hypoxia-inducible factor 1 is a basic-helix-loop-helix-PAS heterodimer regulated by cellular O_2 tension. Proceedings of the National Academy of Sciences of the United States of America. 1995;**92**(12):5510-5514

[17] Rowlands JC, Gustafsson JA. Aryl hydrocarbon receptor-mediated signal transduction. Critical Reviews in Toxicology. 1997;**27**(2):109-134

[18] Whitlock JP Jr. Induction of cytochrome P4501A1. Annual Review of Pharmacology and Toxicology. 1999;**39**:103-125

[19] Bradshaw TD, Trapani V, Vasselin DA, Westwell AD. The aryl hydrocarbon receptor in anticancer drug discovery: Friend or foe? Current Pharmaceutical Design. 2002;**8**(27):2475-2490

[20] Khorram O, Garthwaite M, Golos T. Uterine and ovarian aryl hydrocarbon receptor (AHR) and aryl hydrocarbon receptor nuclear translocator (ARNT) mRNA expression in benign and malignant gynaecological conditions. MHR: Basic Science of Reproductive Medicine. 2002;**8**(1):75-80. DOI: 10.1093/molehr/8.1.75

[21] Castro-Rivera E, Wormke M, Safe S. Estrogen and aryl hydrocarbon responsiveness of ECC-1 endometrial cancer cells. Molecular and Cellular Endocrinology. 1999;**150**(1-2):11-21

[22] Rogers JM, Denison MS. Analysis of the antiestrogenic activity of 2,3,7,8-tetrachlorodibenzo-p-dioxin in human ovarian carcinoma BG-1 cells. Molecular Pharmacology. 2002;**61**(6):1393-1403

[23] Rowlands C, Krishnan V, Wang X, Santostefano M, Safe S, Miller WR, et al. Characterization of the aryl hydrocarbon receptor and aryl hydrocarbon responsiveness in human ovarian carcinoma cell lines. Cancer Research. 1993;**53**:1802-1807

[24] Cannon MJ, Debopam G, Gujja S. Signaling circuits and regulation of immune suppression by ovarian tumor-associated macrophages. Vaccines (Basel). 2015;**3**(2):448-466. DOI: 10.3390/vaccines3020448

[25] Safe S, Lee S-O, Jin U-H. Role of the aryl hydrocarbon receptor in carcinogenesis and potential as a drug target. Toxicological Sciences. 2013;**135**(1):1-16. DOI: 10.1093/toxsci/kft128. Advance Access Publication June 14, 2013

[26] Wang K, Li Y, Jiang YZ, Dai CF, Patankar MS, Song JS, et al. An endogenous aryl hydrocarbon receptor ligand inhibits proliferation and migration of human ovarian cancer cells. Cancer Letters. 2013;**340**(1):63-71

[27] Chua MS, Kashiyama E, Bradshaw T, et al. Role of CYP1A1 in modulation of antitumor properties of the novel agent 2-(4-amino-3-methylphenyl)benzothiazole (DF 203, NSC 674495) in human breast cancer cells. Cancer Research. 2000;**60**(18): 5196-5203

[28] Loaiza-Perez AI, Trapani V, Hose C, et al. Aryl hydrocarbon receptor mediates sensitivity of MCF-7 breast cancer cells to antitumor agent 2-(4-Amino-3-methylphenyl) benzothiazole. Molecular Pharmacology. 2002;**61**(1):13-19

[29] Monks A, Harris E, Hose C, et al. Genotoxic profiling of MCF-7 breast cancer cell line elucidates gene expression modifications underlying toxicity of the anticancer drug 2-(4-amino-3-methylphenyl)-5-fluorobenzothiazole. Molecular Pharmacology. 2003;**63**(3):766-772

[30] Trapani V, Patel V, Leong CO, et al. DNA damage and cell cycle arrest induced by 2-(4-amino-3-methylphenyl)-5- fluorobenzothiazole (5F 203, NSC 703786) is attenuated in aryl hydrocarbon receptor deficient MCF-7 cells. British Journal of Cancer. 2003;**88**(4):599-605

[31] Hose CD, Hollingshead M, Sausville EA, Monks A. Induction of CYP1A1 in tumor cells by the antitumor agent

2-[4-amino-3-methylphenyl]-5-fluoro-benzothiazole: A potential surrogate marker for patient sensitivity. Molecular Cancer Therapeutics. 2003;**2**(12):1265-1272

[32] Bradshaw TD, Shi DF, Shultz RJ, Paull KD, Kelland L, Wilson A, et al. Influence of 2-(4-aminophenyl) benzothiazoles on growth of human ovarian carcinoma cells in vitro and in vivo. British Journal of Cancer. 1998;**78**:421-442

[33] Loaiza-Perez AI, Kenney S, Boswell J, et al. Aryl hydrocarbon receptor activation of an antitumor aminoflavone: Basis of selective toxicity for MCF-7 breast tumor cells. Molecular Cancer Therapeutics. 2004;**3**(6):715-725

[34] Bradshaw TD, Stevens MFG, Calvert H, Plummer R. Clinical trials: Poster presentations. Abstract B59: Preliminary clinical experiences of phortress: Putative role for c-MET inhibition in antitumor activity. In: AACR-NCI-EORTC International Conference: Molecular Targets and Cancer Therapeutics; Nov 15-19, 2009; Boston, MA. Molecular Cancer Therapeutics. 2009;**8**(12 Supplement). DOI: 10.1158/1535-7163

[35] Bazzi R, Bradshaw TD, Rowlands C, Stevens MFG, Bell D. 2-(4-Amino-3-methylphenyl) -5-fluorobenzothiazole is a ligand and shows species-specific partial agonism of the aryl hydrocarbon receptor. Toxicology and Applied Pharmacology. 2009;**237**:102-110

[36] Bradshaw TD, Bibby MJ, Double JA, Fitchner I, Cooper PA, Alley MC, et al. Preclinical evaluation of amino acid prodrugs of novel antitumor 2-(4-amino-3-methylphenyl) benzothiazoles. Molecular Cancer Therapeutics. 2002;**1**:239-246

[37] Leong C-O, Gaskell M, Martin EA, Heydon RT, Farmer PB, Bibby MC, et al. Antitumour 2-(4-aminophenyl) benzothiazoles generate DNA adducts in sensitive tumour cells in vitro and in vivo. British Journal of Cancer. 2003;**88**:470-477

[38] Bradshaw TD, Chua M-S, Browne HL, Trapani V, Sausville EA, Stevens MFG. In vitro evaluation of amino acid prodrugs of novel antitumour 2-(4-amino-3-methylphenyl) benzothiazoles. British Journal of Cancer. 2002;**86**:1348-1354

[39] Leong C-O, Suggitt M, Swaine MJ, Bibby MC, Stevens MFG, Bradshaw TD. In vitro, in vivo and in silico analyses of the antitumor activity of 2-(4-amino-3-methylphenyl)-5-fluorobenzothiazoles. Molecular Cancer Therapeutics. 2004;**3**:1565-1575

[40] Wang K, Guengerich FP. Bioactivation of fluorinated 2-aryl-benzothiazole antitumor molecules by human cytochrome P450s 1A1 and 2W1 and deactivation by cytochrome P450 2S1. Chemical Research in Toxicology. 2012;**25**:1740-1751

[41] Fichtner I, Monks A, Hose C, Stevens MFG, Bradshaw TD. The experimental antitumor agent phortress and doxorubicin are equiactive against human-derived breast carcinoma xenograft models. Breast Cancer Research and Treatment. 2004;**87**:97-107

[42] Hose CD, Hollingshead M, Sausville EA, Monks A. Induction of CYP1A1 in tumor cells by the antitumor agent 2-[4-amino-3-methylphenyl]-5-fluorobenzothiazole: A potential surrogate marker for patient sensitivity. Molecular Cancer Therapeutics. 2003;**2**:1265-1272

[43] Ziech D, Franco R, Pappa A, Panayiotidis MI. Reactive oxygen species (ROS)-induced genetic and epigenetic alterations in human carcinogenesis. Mutation Research. 2011;**711**:167-173

[44] Tandon VR, Sharma S, Mahajan A, Bardi GH. Oxidative stress: Novel strategy in cancer treatment. JK Science. 2005;7:1-3

[45] Mateescu B, Batista L, Cardon M, Gruosso T, de Feraudy Y, Mariani O, et al. miR-141 and miR-200a act on ovarian tumorigenesis by controlling oxidative stress response. Nature Medicine. 2011;**17**:1627-1635

[46] Zuco V, Zanchi C, Cassinelli G, Lanzi C, Supino R, Pisano C, et al. Induction of apoptosis and stress response in ovarian carcinoma cell lines treated with ST 1926, an atypical retinoid. Cell Death and Differentiation. 2004;**11**:280-289

[47] Bradshaw TD, Stone EL, Trapani V, Leong C-O, Matthews CS, te Poele R, et al. Mechanisms of acquired resistance to 2-(4-amino-3-methylphenyl) benzothiazole in breast cancer cell lines. Breast Cancer Research and Treatment. 2008;**110**:57-68

[48] Callero M, Luzzani G, De Dios D, Bradshaw T, Loaiza Perez A. Biomarkers of sensitivity to potent and selective antitumor 2-(4-amino-3-methylphenyl)-5-fluorobenzothiazole (5F203) in ovarian cancer. Journal of Cellular Biochemistry. 2013;**114**(10):2392-2404. DOI: 10.1002/jcb.24589

[49] Vibhuti A, Arif E, Mishra A, Deepak D, Singh B, Rahman I, et al. CYP1A1, CYP1A2, and CYBA gene polymorphisms associated with oxidative stress in COPD. Clinica Chimica Acta. 2010;**411**:474-480

[50] Morgan MJ, Liu Z. Crosstalk of reactive oxygen species and NF-kB signaling. Cell Research. 2011;**21**:103-115

[51] Rogakou EP, Nieves-Neira W, Boon C, Pommier Y, Bonner WM. Initiation of DNA fragmentation during apoptosis induces phosphorylation of H2AX histone at serine 139. The Journal of Biological Chemistry. 2000;**275**:9390-9395

[52] Vathipadiekal V, Saxena D, Mok SC, Hauschka PV, Ozbun L, Birrer MJ. Identification of a potential ovarian cancer stem cell gene expression profile from advanced stage papillary serous ovarian cancer. PLoS One. 2012;7(1):e29079. DOI: 10.1371/journal.pone.0029079

[53] Hutchinson I, Chua M-S, Browne HL, Trapani V, Bradshaw TD, Westwell AD, et al. The synthesis and in vitro biological properties of fluorinated 2-(4-aminophenyl)benzothiazoles. Journal of Medicinal Chemistry. 2001;**44**:1446-1455

[54] Rhoda Lee C. Drug interactions and hormonal contraception. Trends in Urology Gynaecology & Sexual Health May/June 2009. DOI: http://dx.doi.org/10.1002/tre.107

[55] Santes-Palacios R, Romo-Mancillas A, Camacho-Carranza R, Espinosa-Aguirre JJ. Inhibition of human and rat CYP1A1 enzyme by grapefruit juice compounds. Toxicology Letters. Sep 6, 2016;**258**:267-275. DOI: 10.1016/j.toxlet.2016.07.023. Epub 2016 Jul 18

[56] Casper RF, Quesne M, Rogers IM, Shirota T, Jolivet A, Milgrom E, Savouret JF. Resveratrol has antagonist activity on the aryl hydrocarbon receptor: implications for prevention of dioxin toxicity. Molecular Pharmacology. Oct 1999;**56**(4):784-790. https://www.ncbi.nlm.nih.gov/pubmed/10496962

[57] Hestermann EV, Brown M. Agonist and chemopreventative ligands induce differential transcriptional cofactor recruitment by aryl hydrocarbon receptor. Molecular and Cellular Biology. 2003;**23**:7920-7925

[58] Ma Q, Baldwin KT. 2,3,7,8-tetrachloro-dibenzo-p-dioxin-degradation of the

aryl hydrocarbon receptor (AhR) by the ubiquitin proteosome-pathway. The Journal of Biological Chemistry. 2000;**275**:8432-8438

[59] Ikuta T, Eguchi H, Tachibana T, Yoneda Y, Kawajiri K. Nuclear localization and export signals of the human aryl hydrocarbon receptor. The Journal of Biological Chemistry. 1998;**273**:2895-2904

[60] Rowlands CJ, Staskal DF, Gollapudi B, Budinsky R. The human AHR: Identification of single nucleotide polymorphisms from six ethnic populations. Pharmacogenetics and Genomics. 2010;**20**:283-290

[61] Zheng Q, Sha X, Liu J, Heath E, Lorusso P, Li J. Association of human cytochrome P450 1A1 (CYP1A1) and sulfotransferase 1A1 (SULT1A1) polymorphisms with differential metabolism and cytotoxicity of aminoflavone. Molecular Cancer Therapeutics. 2010;**9**:2803-2813

[62] Lin X, Li Q, Wang YJ, Ju YW, Chi ZQ, Wang MW, et al. Morphine inhibits doxorubicin-induced reactive oxygen species generation and nuclear factor kappaB transcriptional activation in neuroblastoma SH-SY5Y cells. The Biochemical Journal. 2007;**406**:215-221

[63] McLean L, Davis W Jr, Sowers E, Brantley EJ. 5F 203-Induced Apoptosis Involves Oxidative Stress and Caspase Activation in Sensitive Breast Cancer Cells. Washington DC, USA: American Association for Cancer Research; 2006

[64] Righetti SC, Perego P, Corna E, Pierotti MA, Zunino F. Emergence of p53 mutant cisplatin-resistant ovarian carcinoma cells following drug exposure: Spontaneously mutant selection. Cell Growth & Differentiation. 1999;**10**:473-478

[65] Assinelli G, Supino R, Perego P, Polizzi D, Lanzi C, Pratesi G, et al. A role for loss of p53 function in sensitivity of ovarian carcinoma cells to taxanes. International Journal of Cancer. 2001;**92**:738-747

[66] Perego P, Giarola M, Righetti SC, Supino R, Caserini C, Delia D, et al. Association between cisplatin resistance and mutation of p53 gene and reduced bax expression in ovarian carcinoma cell systems. Cancer Research. 1996;**56**:556-562

Chapter 6

Functions of miRNAs in the Development, Diagnosis, and Treatment of Ovarian Carcinoma

Hulya Yazici

Abstract

miRNAs (miRNA) are small RNA molecules that are not to expressed to proteins. Their size is 20–22 nucleotides in length and they are highly conserved molecules among the species. miRNAs are synthesized in the nucleus as a primary miRNA. Primary miRNA is transferred to cytoplasm by Xpo5 protein (exportin-5) and then is processed by Dicer enzyme to a 22-nucleotide-sized long mature miRNA. miRNAs are differentially expressed in different diseases and are released into plasma by normal and tumor tissues during the cell metabolism. Ovarian carcinoma is the deadliest cancer among women. When the disease was diagnosed, the disease usually progressed. Currently, there is no biological marker to detect ovarian carcinoma at an early stage. Furthermore, there is a need for markers that are sensitive to chemotherapy changes and early detection of the disease. Because of this, miRNAs can be detected in plasma and can be used as highly significant biological markers and therapeutic targets for ovarian carcinoma. When the literature of the last 5 years is searched, there are many studies about miRNA and ovarian carcinoma. In this chapter, studies examining the relationship between ovarian carcinoma and miRNA from different angles are summarized under different sections.

Keywords: miRNAs, ovarian carcinoma, diagnosis and treatment

1. Introduction

Ovarian cancer (OC) is the sixth common cancer in women in the United States. According to GLOBOCAN data published in 2018, 295,414 new cases of ovarian cancer have been reported in the world. A total of 184,799 of these cases have been reported to have died due to ovarian carcinoma. The patients who died because of ovarian carcinoma had constituted 62.5% of the cases diagnosed in 2018 [1]. Ovarian carcinoma is diagnosed in women at peri- and postmenopausal status frequently [2].

Genetics, syndromes (breast and ovarian carcinoma syndrome and Lynch syndrome), family history, personal history of cancer or endometriosis, increasing age, reproductive history and infertility, hormone replacement therapy, and obesity are factors that may increase the risk of ovarian carcinoma. However, oral contraceptive usage, having pregnancy before age 26, breastfeeding, removal of the ovaries and fallopian tubes, hysterectomy, and tubal ligation are factors that may reduce the risk of ovarian carcinoma. Ovarian carcinoma comprises a heterogeneous group of

IntechOpen

tumors with different histologic subtypes which have particular genetic structures and different response to treatment. The most common histological subtype is epithelial ovarian carcinomas accounting for about 90% of cases and can be classified as serous, endometrioid, and clear-cell and mucinous carcinomas [3, 4].

However, a majority of women are diagnosed in an advanced stage because of the asymptomatic issue in the early stage and due to the lack of an adequate early detection screening method [5]. Ovarian cancer still remains as one of the leading causes of cancer-related deaths, and the treatments could be improved using predictive biomarkers to measure a response to ovarian cancer therapy. Currently, there is no available proven single biomarker in the clinical use for detecting ovarian carcinoma in the early stage with adequate sensitivity and specificity. To solve this problem, researchers have aimed at the identification and validation of novel biomarkers for the early detection of ovarian carcinoma using new technologies. Diagnostic markers for population screening would be a simple blood testing with 95% specificity and sensitivity.

Similar to regulatory RNAs, microRNAs (miRNAs) are frequently deregulated in carcinogenesis. In ovarian tumorigenesis, numerous miRNAs were found altered, and some of these genes might represent ideal targets for diagnosis, prognosis, and treatment [6].

This chapter will focus on the recent advancements in miRNAs in the diagnosis, prognosis, and the treatments resistant to ovarian carcinoma.

2. Methods

PubMed search was performed using the keywords "ovarian carcinoma and miRNA" to prepare a comprehensive literature review. The results were filtered by published manuscripts in the last 5 years. A total of 193 associated papers, and review articles were found in the initial search. Additional searches were performed using the keywords genetic markers in ovarian cancer, multidrug resistance in ovarian cancer, and prognostic markers to supplement the information. 180 papers were selected for inclusion in the manuscript following the careful review of the abstracts. This chapter was written using the data of 3 meta-analyses, 20 reviews, and 67 original papers published in the last 5 years.

3. Biogenesis and functions of miRNAs

MicroRNAs (miRNAs) are a class of small noncoding RNA molecules which regulate gene expression at the posttranscriptional level [7, 8]. Thousands of miRNA sequences have been identified in a wide range of organisms after the discovery of small noncoding RNAs [9, 10] and have currently been shown to be highly conserved among a wide range of species [11]. The miRNA database contains 38,589 entries representing hairpin precursor miRNAs, expressing 48,885 mature miRNA for 271 species (http://microrna.sanger.ac.uk). Each miRNA directly or indirectly regulates approximately 100 mRNA transcripts; however, a single gene coding protein could be regulated by more than one miRNA.

MicroRNAs are transcribed by RNA polymerase II or III, generating primary transcripts as short RNA hairpin structures (pre-miRNA) which are subsequently processed by cytoplasmic RNase III-type enzymes, Drosha and Dicer. The processed, mature miRNA incorporates into the RNA-induced silencing protein complex (RISC) to regulate the function of genes through degradation of mRNA and inhibition of translation [12, 13]. RISC usually binds to the 3′-UTR region of target mRNAs to repress translation. The degree of translation depends on the degree of complementarity between miRNA and target mRNA. miRNAs usually bind to specific sequences with partial complementarity on target RNA transcripts, called microRNA response elements (MREs), which result in translational repression in humans [14, 15].

MicroRNAs were shown to have a crucial function in oncogenesis by regulating cell proliferation, cell differentiation, and apoptosis as oncogenes or tumor suppressors. The deregulation of miRNAs was suggested to be involved in a mechanism for cancer development. Also, miRNAs have been used as potential diagnostic or therapeutic targets in cancer treatment.

3.1 Important miRNAs as diagnostic and prognostic biomarkers and therapeutic targets in ovarian carcinoma

Ovarian carcinoma is the most lethal cancer among gynecological malignancies. Therefore, there is still a need for good diagnostic markers to detect the disease at an early stage and good prognostic markers to follow the effects of therapeutic agents during the chemotherapy of patients with ovarian carcinoma. Li et al. investigated the miR-193b expression level in the tissues of patients diagnosed with ovarian carcinoma and ovarian carcinoma cell lines. They found the aberrant expression level of miR-193b in the tissue of ovarian carcinoma patients. miR-193b showed decreased expression in tumor tissues of patients with ovarian carcinoma and was correlated with FIGO stage, histologic grade, ascites, lymph node metastasis, tumor size, and also poor survival. Therefore, they suggested that the level of miR193b expression could be a potential biomarker for ovarian carcinoma patients [16]. Fukagawa et al. investigated the expression level of miR-135a-3p in the serum of ovarian carcinoma patients compared to ovarian cysts and normal ovarian tissue and also analyzed the expression level of miR-135a-3p in ovarian carcinoma cell lines such as SKOV3, ES2, and xenograft under cisplatin and paclitaxel. According to their result, they suggested that the miR-135a-3p expression could be used as a noninvasive biomarker in serum of patients with ovarian carcinoma in the diagnosis and follow-up of the disease [17]. Zuberi et al. evaluated the impact of the miR-125b expression level in patients with ovarian carcinoma and found that the expression level of miR-125b was statistically significant and that it was increased in serum specimens of patients with ovarian carcinoma compared to the levels in serum specimens of the healthy controls. They also demonstrated that the upregulation of miR-125b was associated with FIGO stage and lymph node involvement and distant metastasis and was correlated with hypermethylation of some tumor suppressor genes such as p16, p14, BRCA1, DAPK1, PTEN, and RASSF1A. Their results suggested that the expression level of mi-125b might be an early diagnostic biomarker to predict distant metastasis and lymph node status [18]. Zhang et al. investigated miR-613 expression in tissue of patients with ovarian carcinoma compared to matched normal adjacent tissue of patients. They found that low expression of miR-613 was associated with the FIGO stage, tumor grade, lymph node involvement, short progression-free survival (PFS), and overall survival (OS) in ovarian carcinoma patients. Their results indicated that miR-613 might be a good prognostic biomarker in patients with retinoblastoma [19]. Yanaihara et al. searched five miRNAs such as miR-132, miR-9, miR-126, miR-34a, and miR-21 in 12 high-grade serous ovarian carcinoma and 15 clear-cell ovarian carcinoma patients. They found that five miRNAs showed statistically higher expression in patients with clear-cell ovarian carcinoma. They also investigated further biological significance of miR-9 expression especially and demonstrated that miR-9 might have distinguished histologic subtypes of ovarian carcinoma and might be used a therapeutic target for treatment of ovarian carcinoma [20]. Yang et al. showed that miR-506 was associated with poor prognosis in ovarian carcinoma (OC) patients [21]. Sun et al. demonstrated in their study that miR-506 expression was correlated with early FIGO stage and good and longer survival [22]. The results of both studies suggested that miR-506 might be used as a prognostic biomarker. Yuan et al. showed that miR-494 had an antitumor effect in the tissue of OC patients and that miR-494 suppressed the cell proliferation and cell migration in epithelial ovarian carcinoma through the c-myc gene [23].

Agostini et al. studied 155 tissues of ovarian carcinoma including 30 sex cord-stromal tumors, 22 borderline tumors, and 103 ovarian carcinomas and investigated the HMGA2 gene and its two miRNA targets in the study. They found that let-7a and miR-30c were highly decreased in all tumors in the study. Their results showed that Let-7a and miR30c were deregulated in OC patients, and the cause of deregulation in let-7a and miR30c might be due to the genomic imbalances, and the genomic imbalances resulted with the upregulation of HMGA2 gene. They suggested further research to better understand the associations between genetic imbalance and miRNA expression and prognostic and diagnostic importance in ovarian carcinoma [24]. Ma et al. investigated the expression level of miR-486-5p and its target, OLFM4 gene. Their results suggested that the decreased expression level of OLFM4 was associated with higher-grade FIGO tumors and poor differentiation. OLFM4 is downregulated by miR-486-5p which contributed to the tumorigenesis of ovarian carcinoma, and the opposite might be possible. OLFM4 and miR-485-5p might be the therapeutic targets for ovarian carcinoma [25]. Teng et al. published an article explaining an association between DNMT3A/3B and miR-29b. The results showed that the downregulation of miR29b was controlled by high levels of DNMT3A/3B expression. The results were suggested that was a cross talk and feedback between DNMT3A/3B and miR-29b and that the expression of miR-29b negatively controlled DNMTs, especially DNMT3A/3B. The findings showed that miR-29b and inhibitors of DNMT3A/B might be therapeutic target for patients with ovarian carcinoma [26]. According to articles published by different authors, miR-199 was downregulated in epithelial ovarian carcinoma and targeted to c-Met, HIF1-alpha, HIF2-beta, and IKK-beta proteins. Therefore, c-Met and/or miR-199 might be a target for patients with metastatic ovarian carcinoma [27–29]. Although many studies have been conducted so far, there are many candidate molecules that can be used in the diagnosis and prognosis of ovarian cancer; however, most of them should be validated with larger patient groups.

3.2 miRNAs responsible for drug resistance in treatment of ovarian carcinoma

The response of a patient with ovarian cancer to chemotherapy is actually the most important factor determining the survival of the patient. The primary treatment for ovarian cancer is surgery. After surgery, the first-line treatment is platinum-based combination [cisplatin or carboplatin and/or taxane (paclitaxel)] [30]. The majority of patients, almost 70%, receive this treatment and show complete remission. Patients were extremely sensitive to chemotherapy when they first received the treatment, and this situation changed during the next relapse period. The pharmacokinetics and pharmacodynamics of platinum-based therapies are known to be influenced by germ line genetic factors [31].

It is stated that many events associated with cisplatin resistance may be effective. It has been thought that these mechanisms can be generated by genetic and epigenetic alterations and miRNAs [32]. It is known that women with BRCA1 and BRCA2 gene mutations had better response to chemotherapy and had longer survival. It was reported that the mechanism underlying situation was associated with miR-9 in animal models. miR-9 downregulates the BRCA1 gene, causing the DNA repair mechanism not to function, and thus increases the sensitivity to chemotherapy. In a study by Sun et al., It was shown that miR-9 overexpression in 58 tumor tissue samples was associated with BRCA1 gene mutation. Accordingly, these patients have been reported to be extremely sensitive to chemotherapy, especially platinum-based drugs and PARP inhibitors [33]. Furthermore, a similar relationship between BRCA1-miR-9 is present between the miR-93 and the PTEN gene. High miR-93 and low PTEN expressions were investigated in ovarian carcinoma cell lines which were OVCAR3 and SKOV3 with and without platinum resistance. In this study by Fu et al., the relationship between PTEN-miR-93 was also shown in tumor tissues of 10 ovarian cancer patients [34]. Let-7 expression has been reported to play a role in the response to chemotherapy. In particular, when paclitaxel was added to platinum regimen, it was shown that chemotherapy is beneficial in patients with low expression of let-7 [35]. It has been reported that high-level expression of miR622 is responsible for the development of resistance to platinum drugs and PARP inhibitors in patients with high-grade serous ovarian cancer with BRCA1 mutation. It is emphasized that this effect of miR622 can be affected by correcting the disorders in the homologous recombination mechanism [36]. The blockade of PD-L1, PD-1, and CTLA-4, which are immune system inhibitor receptors, has been extremely successful in some advanced cancers. High expression of miR-424 (322), especially in tumors, prolongs progression-free survival in ovarian cancer patients. miR-424 (322) blocks PD-L1 and CD80 expressions. The expression of miR424 (322) with PD-L1 immune checkpoint inhibitors is corrected, i.e., it is converted to normal. In in vivo and in vitro conditions, the restoration of miR424 (322), i.e., normalization, eliminates the resistance to chemotherapy by activation of the T cell immune response via blocking PD-L1. There is a synergetic development of chemotherapy and immunotherapy. PD-L1 and chemoresistance are controlled via miRNAs [37]. In the literature, there are a number of studies showing the relationship between miRNAs and chemosensitivity and chemoresistance. Some miRNAs have a highly significant role in the use of combined therapies such as chemotherapy and immunotherapy. There is no doubt that the success of cancer treatments will increase as the relationship between miRNA molecules and cancer treatments is determined. However, there is no doubt that more studies should be done to use these molecules as standard in the clinic.

3.3 Important polymorphisms and mutations of miRNA processing and binding sites in ovarian carcinoma

3.3.1 3′UTR miRNA binding site of the KRAS gene

In 2008, Ratner et al. identified a germ line SNP in 3′UTR of the KRAS oncogene (rs61764370). The functional KRAS-variant was disrupted by the binding of let-7 to 3′UTR region of KRAS gene [38]. In 2010, Ratner et al. reported that a single nucleotide polymorphism (SNP), rs61764370, located in the 3′UTR of the *KRAS* oncogene was associated with the risk of unselected epithelial ovarian cancer [39]. They also showed that the variant was associated with hereditary ovarian cancer patients carrying *BRCA1* mutations and ovarian cancer patients with family history not carrying *BRCA1* or *BRCA2* [39]. This SNP was thought to be a strong candidate for cancer risk. These observations suggested that miRNAs can function as tumor suppressors or oncogenes [40]. An assay has subsequently been marketed to determine genotype at rs61764370 as a commercial test to determine the risk in women with a family history of ovarian cancer (http://www.miradx.com). However, in June 2011, Pharoah et al. showed in an extensive study with 8.669 unselected cases of invasive epithelial ovarian cancer and 10.012 controls that the SNP was clinically useless for risk prediction in sporadic or familial ovarian cancer [41].

3.3.2 3′UTR miRNA binding site of the BRCA1 and BRCA2

BRCA1/2 mutations and targeted miRNAs to BRCA genes were demonstrated in many studies in the last decade [42] [43–45]. Moskwa et al. suggested that tumors overexpressing miRNAs such as miR-182 which target BRCA proteins can also be susceptible to PARP inhibition.

They suggested that the high level of miR-182 expression may affect BRCA1 regulation for sporadic breast tumors. The changing level of miR-182 expression in different types of breast tumor cell lines affected the level of protein expression of BRCA1 and changed the sensitivity to PARP1 inhibition, both in breast cancer cell lines and in xenograft models [42]. Bioinformatic tools showed a binding site for miR-146a and miR-146b-5p in the upstream of BRCA1. This information suggested that BRCA1 gene can be downregulated by miR-146a and miR-146b-5p in basal-like breast cancer cell lines and triple-negative breast tumors. This downregulation of BRCA1 increased a cell proliferation and a reduced homologous recombination repair rate controlled by BRCA1. Garcia et al. showed that the highest levels of miR-146a and/or miR-146b-5p were found in basal-like epithelial mammary tumor cell lines and breast tumors with triple-negative histology, and also the characteristics of these types of tumors are the closest tumors having carriers of BRCA1 mutations [43–45]. miRNAs are known to regulate tumor suppressor genes and oncogenes. The genetic alterations in the binding sites of miRNAs on DNA sequence of miRNA could affect the expression of tumor suppressor genes and oncogenes. Shen et al. searched the selected 17 miRNAs which have an important role in the development of breast cancer in 42 patients with familial breast carcinoma. miR-30c-1 and miR-17 among 17 miRNAs were only observed in noncarriers of BRCA1/2 mutations. They showed that these two miRNAs, miR-30c-1 and miR-17, resulted in conformational changes in their secondary structures and altered the expression in functional assays. They also showed that miR-17 could bind to the 3′UTR of BRCA1 mRNAs. Their results suggested that functional genetic alterations in miRNA genes can potentially alter the regulation of BRCA1 gene which is important for breast cancer [45]. The same perspective and scenario may be valid for patients with sporadic ovarian carcinoma having an overexpression of BRCA1, and the effect of PARP inhibitors can also be increased by eliminating BRCA expression via miR182 in ovarian carcinoma.

3.4 miRNAs as angiogenetic and metastatic biomarkers in ovarian carcinoma

The major challenge in treatment of ovarian carcinoma is the lack of good diagnostic and prognostic factors to follow and to diagnose in each stage of the disease. Li et al. established the study using SKOV3 and OVCAR3 ovarian carcinoma cell lines. They demonstrated that miR-125a-5p, miR125b-5p, miR22-3p, miR205-5p, and miR-152 were significantly downregulated in SKOV3 cell lines and also showed the negative correlation between miR-152 and expression level of ERBB3. The findings of the study showed that miR-152 was associated with the regulation of the proliferation and metastasis of ovarian cancer cells via the repression of ERBB3 expression. miR-152 is an important molecule to suppress the proliferation, invasion, and migration of ovarian carcinoma cell lines. Their results suggested that miR-152 may be a potential therapeutic target for ovarian carcinoma [46].

The interaction between HOTAIR and both miR-214 and miR-217 was shown in the study of Dong et al. on SKOV3 ovarian carcinoma cell line. Their results demonstrated that HOTAIR, which had an interaction with PIK3R3, regulated the proliferation, migration, and invasion in SKOV3 ovarian cell line via miR-214 and miR-217 [47].

Li et al. investigated miR-340 expression in five different ovarian carcinoma cell lines such as OVCAR3, CAOV3, HO-8910, ES-2, A2780, and FTE187. They showed that miR-340 was decreased in ovarian carcinoma cell lines and induced apoptosis in cells with downregulation of NF-ΚB1 to inhibit metastasis in ovarian carcinoma cell lines. They emphasized that miR-340-NF-ΚB1 interaction might be a potential therapeutic target or agent for patients with ovarian carcinoma [48].

Wang et al. examined the expression of MTA1 and miR-30c in ovarian cancer line, SKOV3, and normal human ovarian surface epithelial cell line, HOSE. They found that miR-30c expression was significantly reduced when MTA1 expression was higher and localized in the cytoplasm of the cells. Their results suggested that MTA1 and miR30c expression were altered in ovarian carcinoma cell line and might be associated in invasion and metastasis of patients with ovarian carcinoma [49].

3.5 Important miRNAs in exosomal and peripheral circulations in ovarian carcinoma

Numerous studies demonstrated the clinical importance of circulating miRNAs as diagnostic and prognostic biomarkers in all types of cancer. Circulating miRNAs in ovarian cancer were published in many studies using blood plasma, serum, ascites, and urine.

3.5.1 Exosomal miRNAs

The first study was published by Taylor et al. demonstrating that the levels of eight exosomal microRNAs extracted from sera which were miR-21, miR-141, miR-200a, miR-200c, miR-200b, miR-203, miR-205, and miR-214 were elevated at an advanced-stage ovarian carcinoma [50, 51]. The miRNA signature of exosomes showed that the circulating miRNAs can present the characteristics of the tumor.

3.5.2 miRNAs in sera

Many researchers investigated different miRNAs in the sera of OC patients [51–59].The microRNAs miR182, miR200a, miR200b, and miR200c from miR200 family were investigated by Kan et al. in the sera of OC patients and healthy controls. They found significant differences between patients and controls and suggested that miR200b and miR200c had a power to discriminate serous ovarian cancer from healthy controls and had a potential as a biomarker of sera [53]. Chung et al. showed that the miR-132, miR-26a, miR-let7b, miR-145, and miR-143 were decreased in serum specimens of patients with ovarian carcinoma and healthy individuals [54]. Xu et al. showed significantly higher miR-21 levels in sera of patients with epithelial ovarian cancer than the levels in healthy controls. They also indicated the correlation between the increased miR-21 expression in sera and advanced FIGO stage, high tumor grade, and shortened overall survival. Their findings suggested that serum miR-21 may be a novel diagnostic and prognostic marker and could be used as a therapeutic target in advanced-stage ovarian carcinoma [55]. Hong et al. investigated the serum levels of miR-221 in patients with epithelial ovarian carcinoma and in controls. miR-221 was found to be upregulated in patients with EOC compared with the healthy controls. The expression level of serum miR-221 was significantly associated with the International Federation of Gynecology and Obstetrics (FIGO) stage and tumor grade. In addition, higher serum miR-221 expression was shown to be an independent prognostic factor for epithelial ovarian carcinoma [56].

3.5.3 miRNAs in plasma

Some other scientists used plasma in investigating the circulating biomarkers for ovarian carcinoma [60–63]. Zheng et al. showed higher plasma miR-205 and lower let-7f expression in patients with ovarian carcinoma than in healthy controls. The joint use of both MiR-205 and let-7f provided higher diagnostic accuracy for epithelial ovarian carcinoma, especially in patients with stage I disease. They also demonstrated that the combination of these two miRNAs and carbohydrate antigen-125 (CA-125) further improved the accuracy of detection of epithelial carcinoma in plasma samples and that the elevated miR-483-5p expression was found in patients with ovarian carcinoma with stages III and IV compared with stages I and II. Moreover, they demonstrated that lower levels of let-7f was predictive for poor prognosis in patients with epithelial ovarian carcinoma. Their findings suggested that plasma miR-205 and let-7f can be biomarkers for ovarian cancer detection and prognosis [60]. Shapira et al. assessed the expression levels of 754 miRNAs in presurgical plasma samples of 42 women with serous epithelial ovarian cancer and 36 plasma samples collected from women who had a benign pelvic mass at surgery. There were six miRNAs, miR-106b, miR-126, miR-150, miR-17, miR-20a, and miR-92a which were distinguished as benign in histology before surgery. They showed that 10 miRNAs in plasma can distinguish healthy controls from women with ovarian cancer and a benign neoplasm before surgery. In the comparison of healthy controls with patient's plasma samples, they found that five miRNAs, miR-1274a, miR-30b, miR-30c, miR-625-3p, and miR720, were differentially expressed and also that the level of miR-139-5p, miR-142-3p, miR-484, miR-486, and miR-660 were higher in healthy controls when analyzed against patients having benign mass in their body. They demonstrated that MiR-720 and miR-20a were higher in women who died 2 years after their diagnosis, and women who survived 44 years after diagnosis had higher levels of miR-223, miR-126-3p, and miR-1290 in their plasma before surgery [62].

3.5.4 miRNAs in ascites

Vaksman et al. investigated the effusion supernatants in 86 patients with ovarian carcinoma. In the study, they demonstrated that there were significant associations between clinicopathologic parameters and the levels of miR-21, miR-23a, miR-23b, miR-29a, miR-99a, miR-125b, miR-200c, miR-320a, and miR-484 and also between miRNAs 21, 23b, and 29a and poor survival. It was shown that the higher expression of miR-21 in metastatic ovarian carcinoma constituted chemoresistance in ovarian carcinoma, and the higher expression of miR-23a and miR-29a was associated with significantly shorter PFS [64].

3.5.5 miRNAs in urine

Researchers detected miRNAs on the urine of patients with ovarian carcinoma in the studies in the literature [65, 66]. Zavesky et al. investigated the expression of miRNAs in the urine of patients with ovarian carcinoma and endometrial carcinoma. They compared the expression levels of 18 miRNAs in OC patients before and after surgery. The expression levels of miR-92a, miR100, miR106b, and miR-200b were found significantly different between patients with ovarian carcinoma and healthy controls. The expression levels of miR100 and miR106b were lower; however, the expression levels of miR-92a and miR-200b were higher in patients with ovarian carcinoma compared with the levels in healthy controls [65]. Zhou et al. examined the urine specimen obtained from 39 OC patients, from 26 patients with benign gynecologic disease, and from 30 healthy controls. They found that miR30a-5p was upregulated in OC patients compared with the healthy controls, and they also showed that the level of miR30a-5p can be used to follow excess tissues of ovarian carcinoma after surgery [66].

3.6 Important miRNAs for autophagy in ovarian carcinoma

Some miRNAs participated in the control of autophagy by regulating ATGs proteins [67]. Yang et al. showed that the higher expression of mir-30d regulated autophagy through inhibiting LC3B-I conversion to LC3B-II enzymes and formation of autophagosome. Their results suggested that mir-30d disrupts the process of autophagy targeting multiple genes in the autophagy pathway. The data suggested that miR-30d might participate to oncogenesis and be used in the cancer therapy strategy [68]. Dai et al. investigated the expression levels of miR29b that targeted to genes of myeloid cell leukemia sequence 1 (MCL1), mitogen-activated protein kinase 10 (MAPK10), and autophagy-related protein 9A (ATG9A) and suggested that lower level of miR29b was an independent poor prognostic marker in ovarian carcinoma [69]. He et al. examined the downregulation of ATG14 through EGR1-miR-152 in cisplatin resistance ovarian carcinoma cell lines of A2780, CP70, SKOV3, and DDP. They determined that miR-152 expression level was extremely low in the cisplatin-resistant cell lines. Therefore, they suggested that the overexpression of miR-152 might be a useful therapeutic strategy to overcome cisplatin resistance by inhibiting ATG14 expression in ovarian carcinoma [70].

3.7 Important miRNAs for invasion in ovarian carcinoma

Invasion into surrounding tissue is an important step of metastasis. Therefore, understanding the molecular mechanism of invasion may help to understand the metastasis process and identify novel biomarkers and therapeutic agents to treat and to protect patients against metastasis. Zhang et al. showed that there was a higher expression of miR-630 in 30 patients with ovarian carcinoma [71]. They also showed the effects of higher miR-360 expression in SKOV3 cell line. The results of the cell line study indicated that miR-630 targeted the KLF6 gene (Krüppel-like factor 6). KLF6 gene is responsible for cancer cell proliferation and migration. They demonstrated that miR-630 supported the epithelial cancer proliferation and invasion via targeting KLF6 gene, and overexpression of miR-630 stimulated growth of ovarian carcinoma tumor in vivo. Therefore, miR-630 was suggested to be a possible therapeutic target in ovarian carcinoma [71]. Sun et al. determined that the expression of miR-548c decreased in ovarian and endometrium carcinoma. Their results suggested that miR548c affected the expression of Twist. Higher expression level of Twist was shown in ovarian and endometrium carcinoma. Therefore, they emphasized that miR-548c might be used for therapeutic purposes to impress the expression level of TWIST in overexpressing tumors such as ovarian and endometrium carcinoma [72]. Wei et al. examined miR-205 expression level in 30 patients with ovarian carcinoma and in 12 normal ovarian tissues, and they found miR-205 overexpression in ovarian carcinoma tissue of patients. Also, the behavior of miR-205 was investigated in ovarian carcinoma cell lines of OVCAR5, OVCA8, and SKOV3. They determined that miR205 targeted to TCF21 gene (transcription factor 21) which significantly decreased in tumor tissue of OC patients [73]. They concluded that miR-205 was associated with the invasive behavior of ovarian tumor cells by targeting and with the decrease of TCF21 expression. miR-205 and TCF21 were suggested to be used for anticancer purposes [73]. Human telomerase reverse transcriptase (hTERT) is another important molecule in ovarian carcinoma. Bai et al. investigated expression levels of miR-532 and miR-3064 and found that they were downregulated in 60 tumor tissues of ovarian cancer patients, and there was an association between the decreased miR-532 and miR-3064 and poor survival of patients with ovarian carcinoma. Bai et al. also demonstrated that miR-532 and miR-3064 targeted to hTERT gene and inhibited the proliferation, epithelial-mesenchymal transitions (EMT), and invasion of ovarian carcinoma cells. Their results showed that miR-3064 controlled the expression level of hTERT, and the role of miR-532 was limited in ovarian carcinoma. They suggested that both miR-532 and miR-3064 might be a good therapeutic agent for treatment of ovarian carcinoma [74].

3.8 An impact of miRNAs on epithelial-mesenchymal transitions (EMT) in ovarian carcinoma

3.8.1 miR-125a

The epithelial-to-mesenchymal transition (EMT) and its reversion, mesenchymal-to-epithelial transition (MET), are important mechanisms in carcinoma progression and tumor metastasis. The important regulators of this process are growth factors, transcription factors, and adhesion molecules in that the activity of microRNA (miRNA) is suggested to contribute to EMT, MET, and metastatic progression. In ovarian cancer cells, EMT induces by overexpression of EGFR which leads to transcriptional repression of the miR-125a. MiR125a is suggested to be a negative regulator of EMT. Therefore, the repression of miR-125a was suggested to be a potential novel therapeutic approach for invasive behavior of ovarian cancer [75].

3.8.2 miR-125b

miR-125b expression was lower in epithelial ovarian carcinoma. The expression of miR125b in ovarian carcinoma blocked the tumor invasion. The expression of miR125b was associated with EMT and also with the expression of SET gene. Functional studies showed that SET gene was a target for miR-125b. The downregulated SET gene may be observed during tumor migration [76].

3.8.3 miR-200 family

Various studies on miR-200 family showed that the miR-200 family was associated with the inhibition of cancer metastasis via epithelial-to-mesenchymal transition. mRNAs of SMAD and ZEB gene families are the key targets for the inhibition of cancer cell metastasis stimulated by miR-200 via EMT. ZEB2 has specific sequences on its' 3′ UTR region for miR-200a, miR-141, miR-200b, miR-200c, 429, miR-200a, and miR-141. ZEB1 and ZEB2 are transcriptional repressor of E-Cadherin [77]. Wang et al. determined that the higher expressions of miR-429 and miR-200 families in mesenchymal-like ovarian carcinoma cell lines elevated the MET and the sensitivity to cisplatin [78]. In addition, TET3 was a gene downregulated during the epithelial-mesenchymal transition (EMT) induced with TGF-β1 in ovarian carcinoma cell lines. miR-30d was associated as a downstream target of TET3 gene. miR-30d could not bind to the promoter of TET3 gene, and TGF-β1-associated EMT was stimulated owing to the demethylation on binding site of miR-30d [79].

3.9 Important miRNAs on survival in ovarian carcinoma

Fu et al. found higher miR-222-3p expression level in tumors of OC patients. They determined that the overexpression of miR-222-3p was associated with good survival in patients with epithelial ovarian carcinoma. As a further research, they also investigated biological function of miR-222-3p in cell lines and in mouse models. The data of the in vitro experiments determined that miR-222-3p suppressed the cell proliferation and migration in ovarian cancer cell lines and downregulated AKT activation by decreased phosphorylation of AKT protein. They showed that GNAI2 is a target for miR-222-3p and also induced PI3K/AKT pathway. They suggested that miR222-3p/GNAI2/AKT interactions might be used as a therapeutic target in ovarian carcinoma [80]. Zhou et al. showed that miR-595 is a significant biomarker to show poor prognosis in patients in ovarian carcinoma. They investigated miR-595 in tumors in epithelial ovarian carcinoma, and the lower expression of miR-595 was found associated with advanced FIGO stage and distant metastasis and short overall survival [81]. Shi et al. published a meta-analysis about miR-200 and miR-30. They showed that the expression levels of miR-200 family had significant association with overall survival (OS) and insignificant association with progression-free survival (PFS) in general evaluation. They also evaluated their results in subgroup analysis and found that an increased expression level of miR-200a, miR-200c, and miR-141 was associated with better PFS for patients with ovarian carcinoma. A higher expression level of miR-30 was associated with good overall survival and progression-free survival [82]. Therefore, they suggested that both miR200 family and miR-30 might be good prognostic biomarkers in patients with ovarian carcinoma. Kleeman et al. examined the prognostic and apoptotic potentials of miR-147b, miR-1912, and miR-3073a in ovarian carcinoma cell lines which have different genetic backgrounds such as SKOV3 (TP53 null), OVCAAR3 (TP53R248Q), TOV21G, TOV112D (TP53R175H), A2780, and A2780cis (TP53K351N) with/without adding the chemotherapeutic agent of carboplatin. They showed that the expression level of miR-147b and miR-1912 was higher after carboplatin treatment in ovarian cancer cell lines, while the expression level of miR-147b and miR-1912 was lower in untreated ovarian cancer cell line with carboplatin. They underlined that these two-miRNA were leaded pro apoptotic signals and decreased the expression level of Bcl2 and affected to median survival of ovarian carcinoma cell lines [83]. Yoshioka et al. published that the expression level of WNT7A gene was higher in 300 FFPE tissue of ovarian specimens including ovarian tumor, benign/borderline, and normal ovarian tissue. They used ovarian carcinoma cell lines and mouse models to characterize the role of WNT7A gene in ovarian tumor development and progression. They suggested that the re-expression of WNT7A gene could play an important role in malignant transformation of ovarian tissue and progression of ovarian carcinoma [84]. After the article was published by Yoshioka et al., MacLean et al. demonstrated that miR-15b expression targeted WNT7A gene and found an inverse association between WNT7A and miR-15b. Higher expression level of WNT7A gene and lower expression level of miR-15b were associated with poor survival in patients with ovarian carcinoma. Their data showed that WNT7A was controlled by miR-15b expression reduced by promoter methylation through the DNMT1 gene, a responsible methylation in the genome of ovarian carcinoma [85]. Sun et al. published meta-analysis on miR-9 and its prognostic importance in ovarian carcinoma. Their results revealed that the decreased expression level of miR-9 was found to be associated with poor overall survival (OS) and PFS in patients with ovarian carcinoma [86]. Wang et al. demonstrated that higher level expression of miR-532-5p was associated with the survival of patients with ovarian carcinoma in TCGA data and also ovarian carcinoma cell lines, such as SKOV3 and OVCAR3 [87].

4. Conclusion remarks

Over the last 5 years, a large number of studies have been carried out to reveal the relationship between ovarian carcinoma and miRNAs. All of these studies about miRNA are promising for early detection of ovarian cancer, monitoring treatment, determining chemotherapy resistance, and discovering new therapeutic agents. With more extensive studies in the future and the use of effective miRNA molecules found in the clinic, ovarian cancer will be more manageable and early detectable. There is a need for a large number of well-selected patient groups and validated studies for miRNAs to be involved and used in the routine clinic practice. However, when all studies are completed, it is undoubted that miRNAs will contribute to cancer diagnosis, prognosis, and development of new chemotherapeutic drugs and beneficial to individualized medicine. It will be understood that the effects of these small molecules are actually greater than it is thought in the future.

Author details

Hulya Yazici
Oncology Institute, Department of Basic Oncology, Cancer Genetics Division, Istanbul University, Istanbul, Turkey

*Address all correspondence to: hulyayazici67@gmail.com

References

[1] Bray F et al. Global cancer statistics 2018: GLOBOCAN estimates of incidence and mortality worldwide for 36 cancers in 185 countries. CA: A Cancer Journal for Clinicians. 2018;**68**(6):394-424

[2] Jones MB. Borderline ovarian tumors: Current concepts for prognostic factors and clinical management. Clinical Obstetrics and Gynecology. 2006;**49**(3):517-525

[3] Cho KR, Shih Ie M. Ovarian cancer. Annual Review of Pathology. 2009;**4**:287-313

[4] Seidman JD et al. The histologic type and stage distribution of ovarian carcinomas of surface epithelial origin. International Journal of Gynecological Pathology. 2004;**23**(1):41-44

[5] Jemal A et al. Cancer statistics, 2009. CA: A Cancer Journal for Clinicians. 2009;**59**(4):225-249

[6] Bartels CL, Tsongalis GJ. MicroRNAs: Novel biomarkers for human cancer. Clinical Chemistry. 2009;**55**(4):623-631

[7] Cullen BR. Derivation and function of small interfering RNAs and microRNAs. Virus Research. 2004;**102**(1):3-9

[8] Liu X, Fortin K, Mourelatos Z. MicroRNAs: Biogenesis and molecular functions. Brain Pathology. 2008;**18**(1):113-121

[9] Lee RC, Feinbaum RL, Ambros V. The *C. elegans* heterochronic gene lin-4 encodes small RNAs with antisense complementarity to lin-14. Cell. 1993;**75**(5):843-854

[10] Reinhart BJ et al. The 21-nucleotide let-7 RNA regulates developmental timing in *Caenorhabditis elegans*. Nature. 2000;**403**(6772):901-906

[11] Wheeler BM et al. The deep evolution of metazoan microRNAs. Evolution & Development. 2009;**11**(1):50-68

[12] Bartel DP. MicroRNAs: Genomics, biogenesis, mechanism, and function. Cell. 2004;**116**(2):281-297

[13] Kim VN, Han J, Siomi MC. Biogenesis of small RNAs in animals. Nature Reviews. Molecular Cell Biology. 2009;**10**(2):126-139

[14] Shah MY, Calin GA. MicroRNAs as therapeutic targets in human cancers. Wiley Interdisciplinary Reviews: RNA. 2014;**5**(4):537-548

[15] Bhartiya D, Scaria V. Genomic variations in non-coding RNAs: Structure, function and regulation. Genomics. 2016;**107**(2-3):59-68

[16] Li H et al. Tissue miR-193b as a novel biomarker for patients with ovarian cancer. Medical Science Monitor. 2015;**21**:3929-3934

[17] Fukagawa S et al. MicroRNA-135a-3p as a promising biomarker and nucleic acid therapeutic agent for ovarian cancer. Cancer Science. 2017;**108**(5):886-896

[18] Zuberi M et al. Utility of serum miR-125b as a diagnostic and prognostic indicator and its alliance with a panel of tumor suppressor genes in epithelial ovarian cancer. PLoS One. 2016;**11**(4):e0153902

[19] Zhang X, Zhang H. Diminished miR-613 expression as a novel prognostic biomarker for human ovarian cancer. European Review for Medical and Pharmacological Sciences. 2016;**20**(5):837-841

[20] Yanaihara N et al. MicroRNA gene expression signature driven

by miR-9 overexpression in ovarian clear cell carcinoma. PLoS One. 2016;**11**(9):e0162584

[21] Yang D et al. Integrated analyses identify a master microRNA regulatory network for the mesenchymal subtype in serous ovarian cancer. Cancer Cell. 2013;**23**(2):186-199

[22] Sun Y et al. MiR-506 inhibits multiple targets in the epithelial-to-mesenchymal transition network and is associated with good prognosis in epithelial ovarian cancer. The Journal of Pathology. 2015;**235**(1):25-36

[23] Yuan J, Wang K, Xi M. MiR-494 inhibits epithelial ovarian cancer growth by targeting c-Myc. Medical Science Monitor. 2016;**22**:617-624

[24] Agostini A et al. Expressions of miR-30c and let-7a are inversely correlated with HMGA2 expression in squamous cell carcinoma of the vulva. Oncotarget. 2016;**7**(51):85058-85062

[25] Ma H et al. Estrogen receptor-mediated miR-486-5p regulation of OLFM4 expression in ovarian cancer. Oncotarget. 2016;**7**(9):10594-10605

[26] Teng Y et al. A double-negative feedback interaction between MicroRNA-29b and DNMT3A/3B contributes to ovarian cancer progression. Cellular Physiology and Biochemistry. 2016;**39**(6):2341-2352

[27] Kinose Y et al. The hypoxia-related microRNA miR-199a-3p displays tumor suppressor functions in ovarian carcinoma. Oncotarget. 2015;**6**(13):11342-11356

[28] Joshi HP et al. Dynamin 2 along with microRNA-199a reciprocally regulate hypoxia-inducible factors and ovarian cancer metastasis. Proceedings of the National Academy of Sciences of the United States of America. 2014;**111**(14):5331-5336

[29] Chen R et al. Regulation of IKKbeta by miR-199a affects NF-kappaB activity in ovarian cancer cells. Oncogene. 2008;**27**(34):4712-4723

[30] Pignata S et al. Chemotherapy in epithelial ovarian cancer. Cancer Letters. 2011;**303**(2):73-83

[31] Permuth-Wey J et al. STAT3 polymorphisms may predict an unfavorable response to first-line platinum-based therapy for women with advanced serous epithelial ovarian cancer. International Journal of Cancer. 2016;**138**(3):612-619

[32] Cao J et al. DNA methylation-mediated repression of miR-886-3p predicts poor outcome of human small cell lung cancer. Cancer Research. 2013;**73**(11):3326-3335

[33] Sun C et al. miR-9 regulation of BRCA1 and ovarian cancer sensitivity to cisplatin and PARP inhibition. Journal of the National Cancer Institute. 2013;**105**(22):1750-1758

[34] Fu X et al. Involvement of microRNA-93, a new regulator of PTEN/Akt signaling pathway, in regulation of chemotherapeutic drug cisplatin chemosensitivity in ovarian cancer cells. FEBS Letters. 2012;**586**(9):1279-1286

[35] Iorio MV, Croce CM. Commentary on microRNA fingerprint in human epithelial ovarian cancer. Cancer Research. 2016;**76**(21):6143-6145

[36] Choi YE et al. Platinum and PARP inhibitor resistance due to overexpression of MicroRNA-622 in BRCA1-mutant ovarian cancer. Cell Reports. 2016;**14**(3):429-439

[37] Xu S et al. miR-424(322) reverses chemoresistance via T-cell immune response activation by blocking the PD-L1 immune checkpoint. Nature Communications. 2016;**7**:11406

[38] Chin LJ et al. A SNP in a let-7 microRNA complementary site in the KRAS 3′ untranslated region increases non-small cell lung cancer risk. Cancer Research. 2008;**68**(20):8535-8540

[39] Ratner E et al. A KRAS-variant in ovarian cancer acts as a genetic marker of cancer risk. Cancer Research. 2010;**70**(16):6509-6515

[40] Esquela-Kerscher A, Slack FJ. Oncomirs—MicroRNAs with a role in cancer. Nature Reviews. Cancer. 2006;**6**(4):259-269

[41] Pharoah PD et al. The role of KRAS rs61764370 in invasive epithelial ovarian cancer: Implications for clinical testing. Clinical Cancer Research. 2011;**17**(11):3742-3750

[42] Moskwa P et al. miR-182-mediated downregulation of BRCA1 impacts DNA repair and sensitivity to PARP inhibitors. Molecular Cell. 2011;**41**(2):210-220

[43] Garcia AI et al. Down-regulation of BRCA1 expression by miR-146a and miR-146b-5p in triple negative sporadic breast cancers. EMBO Molecular Medicine. 2011;**3**(5):279-290

[44] Shen J et al. A functional polymorphism in the miR-146a gene and age of familial breast/ovarian cancer diagnosis. Carcinogenesis. 2008;**29**(10):1963-1966

[45] Shen J, Ambrosone CB, Zhao H. Novel genetic variants in microRNA genes and familial breast cancer. International Journal of Cancer. 2009;**124**(5):1178-1182

[46] Li LW et al. miR-152 is involved in the proliferation and metastasis of ovarian cancer through repression of ERBB3. International Journal of Molecular Medicine. 2018;**41**(3):1529-1535

[47] Dong L, Hui L. HOTAIR promotes proliferation, migration, and invasion of ovarian cancer SKOV3 cells through regulating PIK3R3. Medical Science Monitor. 2016;**22**:325-331

[48] Li P, Sun Y, Liu Q. MicroRNA-340 induces apoptosis and inhibits metastasis of ovarian cancer cells by inactivation of NF-x03BA;B1. Cellular Physiology and Biochemistry. 2016;**38**(5):1915-1927

[49] Wang X et al. MicroRNA-30c inhibits metastasis of ovarian cancer by targeting metastasis-associated gene 1. Journal of Cancer Research and Therapeutics. 2017;**13**(4):676-682

[50] Taylor DD, Gercel-Taylor C. MicroRNA signatures of tumor-derived exosomes as diagnostic biomarkers of ovarian cancer. Gynecologic Oncology. 2008;**110**(1):13-21

[51] Zuberi M et al. Expression of serum miR-200a, miR-200b, and miR-200c as candidate biomarkers in epithelial ovarian cancer and their association with clinicopathological features. Clinical & Translational Oncology. 2015;**17**(10):779-787

[52] Resnick KE et al. The detection of differentially expressed microRNAs from the serum of ovarian cancer patients using a novel real-time PCR platform. Gynecologic Oncology. 2009;**112**(1):55-59

[53] Kan CW et al. Elevated levels of circulating microRNA-200 family members correlate with serous epithelial ovarian cancer. BMC Cancer. 2012;**12**:627

[54] Chung YW et al. Detection of microRNA as novel biomarkers of epithelial ovarian cancer from the serum of ovarian cancer patients. International Journal of Gynecological Cancer. 2013;**23**(4):673-679

[55] Xu YZ et al. Identification of serum microRNA-21 as a biomarker for early detection and prognosis in human epithelial ovarian cancer. Asian Pacific Journal of Cancer Prevention. 2013;**14**(2):1057-1060

[56] Hong F et al. Prognostic significance of serum microRNA-221 expression in human epithelial ovarian cancer. The Journal of International Medical Research. 2013;**41**(1):64-71

[57] Meng X et al. Diagnostic and prognostic potential of serum miR-7, miR-16, miR-25, miR-93, miR-182, miR-376a and miR-429 in ovarian cancer patients. British Journal of Cancer. 2015;**113**(9):1358-1366

[58] Gao YC, Wu J. MicroRNA-200c and microRNA-141 as potential diagnostic and prognostic biomarkers for ovarian cancer. Tumour Biology. 2015;**36**(6):4843-4850

[59] Liang H et al. Serum microRNA-145 as a novel biomarker in human ovarian cancer. Tumour Biology. 2015;**36**(7):5305-5313

[60] Zheng H et al. Plasma miRNAs as diagnostic and prognostic biomarkers for ovarian cancer. PLoS One. 2013;**8**(11):e77853

[61] Suryawanshi S et al. Plasma microRNAs as novel biomarkers for endometriosis and endometriosis-associated ovarian cancer. Clinical Cancer Research. 2013;**19**(5):1213-1224

[62] Shapira I et al. Circulating biomarkers for detection of ovarian cancer and predicting cancer outcomes. British Journal of Cancer. 2014;**110**(4):976-983

[63] Langhe R et al. A novel serum microRNA panel to discriminate benign from malignant ovarian disease. Cancer Letters. 2015;**356**(2 Pt B):628-636

[64] Vaksman O et al. Exosome-derived miRNAs and ovarian carcinoma progression. Carcinogenesis. 2014;**35**(9):2113-2120

[65] Zavesky L et al. Evaluation of cell-free urine microRNAs expression for the use in diagnosis of ovarian and endometrial cancers. A pilot study. Pathology Oncology Research. 2015;**21**(4):1027-1035

[66] Zhou J et al. Urinary microRNA-30a-5p is a potential biomarker for ovarian serous adenocarcinoma. Oncology Reports. 2015;**33**(6):2915-2923

[67] Titone R et al. Epigenetic control of autophagy by microRNAs in ovarian cancer. BioMed Research International. 2014;**2014**:343542

[68] Yang X et al. mir-30d Regulates multiple genes in the autophagy pathway and impairs autophagy process in human cancer cells. Biochemical and Biophysical Research Communications. 2013;**431**(3):617-622

[69] Dai F, Zhang Y, Chen Y. Involvement of miR-29b signaling in the sensitivity to chemotherapy in patients with ovarian carcinoma. Human Pathology. 2014;**45**(6):1285-1293

[70] He J et al. Downregulation of ATG14 by EGR1-MIR152 sensitizes ovarian cancer cells to cisplatin-induced apoptosis by inhibiting cyto-protective autophagy. Autophagy. 2015;**11**(2):373-384

[71] Zhang S et al. MiR-630 promotes epithelial ovarian cancer proliferation and invasion via targeting KLF6. European Review for Medical and Pharmacological Sciences. 2017;**21**(20):4542-4547

[72] Sun X et al. MiR-548c impairs migration and invasion of endometrial and ovarian cancer cells via downregulation of Twist. Journal

of Experimental & Clinical Cancer Research. 2016;**35**:10

[73] Wei J et al. MicroRNA-205 promotes cell invasion by repressing TCF21 in human ovarian cancer. Journal of Ovarian Research. 2017;**10**(1):33

[74] Bai L et al. MicroRNA-532 and microRNA-3064 inhibit cell proliferation and invasion by acting as direct regulators of human telomerase reverse transcriptase in ovarian cancer. PLoS One. 2017;**12**(3):e0173912

[75] Cowden Dahl KD et al. The epidermal growth factor receptor responsive miR-125a represses mesenchymal morphology in ovarian cancer cells. Neoplasia. 2009;**11**(11):1208-1215

[76] Ying X et al. MicroRNA-125b suppresses ovarian cancer progression via suppression of the epithelial-mesenchymal transition pathway by targeting the SET protein. Cellular Physiology and Biochemistry. 2016;**39**(2):501-510

[77] Park SM et al. The miR-200 family determines the epithelial phenotype of cancer cells by targeting the E-cadherin repressors ZEB1 and ZEB2. Genes & Development. 2008;**22**(7):894-907

[78] Wang L et al. Ectopic over-expression of miR-429 induces mesenchymal-to-epithelial transition (MET) and increased drug sensitivity in metastasizing ovarian cancer cells. Gynecologic Oncology. 2014;**134**(1):96-103

[79] Ye Z et al. TET3 inhibits TGF-beta1-induced epithelial-mesenchymal transition by demethylating miR-30d precursor gene in ovarian cancer cells. Journal of Experimental & Clinical Cancer Research. 2016;**35**:72

[80] Fu X et al. MicroRNA-222-3p/GNAI2/AKT axis inhibits epithelial ovarian cancer cell growth and associates with good overall survival. Oncotarget. 2016;**7**(49):80633-80654

[81] Zhou QH et al. Mir-595 is a significant indicator of poor patient prognosis in epithelial ovarian cancer. European Review for Medical and Pharmacological Sciences. 2017;**21**(19):4278-4282

[82] Shi M et al. MicroRNA-200 and microRNA-30 family as prognostic molecular signatures in ovarian cancer: A meta-analysis. Medicine (Baltimore). 2018;**97**(32):e11505

[83] Kleemann M et al. Investigation on tissue specific effects of pro-apoptotic micro RNAs revealed miR-147b as a potential biomarker in ovarian cancer prognosis. Oncotarget. 2017;**8**(12):18773-18791

[84] Yoshioka S et al. WNT7A regulates tumor growth and progression in ovarian cancer through the WNT/beta-catenin pathway. Molecular Cancer Research. 2012;**10**(3):469-482

[85] MacLean JA 2nd et al. WNT7A regulation by miR-15b in ovarian cancer. PLoS One. 2016;**11**(5):e0156109

[86] Sun H et al. Prognostic value of microRNA-9 in cancers: A systematic review and meta-analysis. Oncotarget. 2016;**7**(41):67020-67032

[87] Wang F et al. High expression of miR-532-5p, a tumor suppressor, leads to better prognosis in ovarian cancer both in vivo and in vitro. Molecular Cancer Therapeutics. 2016;**15**(5):1123-1131

Section 4

Paraneoplastic Syndromes

Chapter 7

Paraneoplastic Pemphigus Is a Life-Threatening Disease

Richard Lucas Konichi-Dias

Abstract

Paraneoplastic pemphigus is a multiorganic autoimmune disease, usually triggered by neoplasias, mainly of lymphoproliferative origin such as chronic lymphocytic leukemia, multiple myeloma, non-Hodgkin's lymphoma, Castleman disease, and thymoma. This disorder is characterized by the presence of autoantibodies that react against proteins, such as desmoplakins, desmocollins, and others existing in cell junctions. The prognosis is reserved, and the mortality rate of the disease is very high, thus proving to be an additional challenge in the therapeutic management of onco-hematological diseases. The objective of this chapter is to solve the main clinical aspects of paraneoplastic pemphigus in lymphoproliferative hematological diseases, anatomopathological and immunofluorescence characteristics, as well as associations with the main differential diagnoses and therapeutic management. We will also describe the main differential diagnoses of paraneoplastic pemphigus, such as various types of pemphigus including induced drug, bullous pemphigoid, drug eruption, lichen planus, graft versus host disease, erythema multiforme, Stevens-Johnson syndrome, and toxic epidermal necrolysis. In addition, the prognosis and quality of life will be mentioned.

Keywords: paraneoplastic pemphigus, neoplasms disease, autoimmune disease

1. Introduction

Paraneoplastic pemphigus (PNP) was first described in 1990 by Anhalt et al. as a rare autoimmune disease that causes ulcerated lesions and vesicular eruptions in the mucocutaneous regions [1]. In 2001, the researcher Nguyen et al. introduced the term multiorganic autoimmune paraneoplastic syndrome, since it is a systemic disease that can affect the kidneys, bladder, and smooth and striated muscles [2]. PNP is a disease triggered mainly by B-cell lymphomas and malignant hematological diseases [3]. Other neoplasms also demonstrate the onset of this disease, as well as carcinoma of the stomach, lung, and colon [3]. The patients with PNP present high mortality rates, being around 90% of the cases, besides presenting an extremely complex and difficult diagnosis, since it resembles several other diseases [4, 5]. The treatment and management of this disease are often ineffective, as it is an extremely aggressive and lethal disease.

In this chapter, we will address the epidemiological aspects, the main triggers, pathophysiology, main manifestations, diagnosis, differential diagnoses, treatments used, prognosis, and the quality of life of patients affected by PNP.

IntechOpen

2. Epidemiology

Because PNP is an extremely rare disease, there is still no data on the incidence of this disease in the world population [3]. To date, about 500 cases have been reported in the literature, with PNP representing 3–5% of all cases of pemphigus in the population [6–8]. The vast majority of affected patients demonstrate lymphoproliferative disorders (LPD) [9]. Although this disease can affect children and adolescents, the most common age group is between 45 and 70 years of age and is not correlated with place of origin, race, and sex [7, 10–14].

3. Association with malignancy and genetic background

PNP can be triggered by several types of neoplasias; however, about 84% of all patients present neoplasias or hematological disorders [3, 7, 15]. Non-Hodgkin's lymphoma is the most common disorder with 38.6% of cases, followed by chronic lymphocytic leukemia and Castleman disease with 18.4% each (**Table 1**). Among the non-hematological neoplasms, sarcomas present approximately 8.6% of the cases, such as leiomyosarcoma, malignant nerve sheath tumor, poorly differentiated sarcoma, reticular cell sarcoma, dendritic cell sarcoma, liposarcoma, and inflammatory myofibroblastoma [15–17]. Other less common diseases described in the literature that provide PNP are malignant thymoma, squamous cell carcinoma of the esophagus, colon carcinoma, CD8+ T-cell lymphoma, retroperitoneal Kaposi's sarcoma, and lymphoepithelioma-like carcinoma [18–23]. Although the PNP is triggered by several neoplasias, the manifestations of this disease may precede the hematological disorders and other malignancies, thus requiring the frequent and continuous follow-up of these patients [15]. In addition, there are reports of the occurrence of PNP without a detecting the cause [24, 25].

It is known that the major histocompatibility complex (MHC) has important relationships in increasing the susceptibility of autoimmune diseases. Although there are few papers that analyze the relationship between PNP and genetics, some studies in the Caucasian and Chinese population showed the relationships of the HLA class II alleles DRB1*03 and HLA-Cw*14 in the PNP's trigger [26, 27]. HLA-Cw* 14 proved to be a more specific allele type of PNP. Its importance has been associated with PNP, regardless of whether it is a Castleman disease or other tumors, in addition to Castleman disease. [26]. However, to date, these studies are preliminary studies that suggest the association between genetic factors and PNP. To better understand this relationship, it is important to conduct studies with larger numbers of patients and that are affected by different tumors, as well as the realization of this association in different populations.

Neoplasms	Frequencies (%)
Non-Hodgkin's lymphoma	38.6
Chronic lymphocytic leukemia	18.4
Castleman disease	18.4
Sarcoma	8.6
Others	16

Table 1.
Paraneoplastic pemphigus associated with neoplasms.

4. Pathogenesis

PNP even being a disease not yet known at the present time, it is known that both autoantibodies, as cell-mediated immunity, are involved [28]. Certainly, it deduces that the immune system is paramount in the pathophysiology of this disease.

4.1 Autoantibodies

PNP triggers immune changes with the production of autoantibodies capable of acting on various proteins in the body. The major target proteins of the autoantibodies are desmoglein 1 (DSG-1) and desmoglein 3 (DSG-3); desmocollins 1, 2, and 3; desmoplakins 1 and 2; BP230; BP130; and envoplakin, in addition to several other epitopes affected by autoantigens found in the individual [29]. These characteristics demonstrate the immunological complexity of the disease.

Proteins of the plakin family, such as desmoplakins 1 and 2, envoplakin, periplakin, plectin and BP230, demonstrate the major targets of autoantibodies [30]. In contrast, the proteins of the cadherin family are the second most affected, with proteins such as DSG-1 and DSG-3 and desmocollin [31]. It is known that the presence of autoantibodies to some proteins are not related to the clinical practice of the patients, although there is a study that has mentioned DSG-3 relation with genital involvement [32].

Other autoantibodies such as alpha-2 macroglobulin-like 1 (A2ML1), a broad-range protease inhibitor, have been shown to be important in some patients. This protein has been shown to increase in the oral mucosa, intestine, esophagus, and muscles. However, its true function in the epithelium is unknown [33, 34].

PNP studies with tumor resection demonstrate that tumors have the capacity to secrete autoantibodies capable of affecting the proteins of the epidermal region [35]. While knowing that most PNPs are involved in neoplastic and LPD diseases, triggering by solid tumors is still poorly understood and demonstrates other mechanisms involved in the production of autoantibodies to plakin proteins.

The involvement of the humoral immunity of PNP presents the desmoplakins 1 and 2, envoplakin, periplakin, BP230, A2ML1, and DSG-1 and DSG-3 as the main proteins of concern [1]. However, 16% of all affected do not demonstrate the presence of these autoantibodies, and this makes, in some cases, the accomplishment of the early diagnosis difficult. A study conducted in patients with PNP and who developed muscle weakness demonstrated autoantibodies against neuromuscular junction proteins and muscle tissue. These muscle-associated proteins were autoantibodies to anti-acetylcholinesterase receptors and anti-titin and anti-ryanodine receptor [36].

4.2 Cellular immunity

Cellular immunity has evidenced important roles in the immunophenotyping of PNP. Pathological analyses have demonstrated inflammatory infiltrates with the presence of CD8+ T cells, CD68+ monocytes, and non-major histocompatibility complex-restricted CD56+ in the subepidermal region [2, 37]. Besides that, in the places of affection, the increase in tumor necrosis factor, as well as interferon gamma, was evidenced [38]. These findings show the importance of cellular immunity in the pathogenesis of the disease, since they present abundantly in the sites of PNP involvement.

5. Clinical features

PNP presents several symptoms and clinical evolutions. The first symptoms as well as the progression of the disease are very varied from one patient to another. However, there are more frequent clinical features of these individuals.

5.1 Oral lesions

The oral mucosa is often affected in patients with PNP [3, 39, 40]. Oral symptoms may be the first symptoms in these patients, even before skin lesions [41]. The most common symptoms are oral and labial erosions with bleeding that may be associated with blisters, macules, papules, vesicles, and erythema (**Figure 1**). In addition, these patients may present a positive Nikolsky sign [41].

PNP lesions may be similar to oral manifestations of other diseases. Pemphigus vulgaris is a disease that initially triggers blisters and ulcers in the oral mucosa (especially on the cheeks) and may even reach the body. Erythema multiforme also affects the region of the oral mucosa with the appearance of erythema, edema, and some superficial erosions with formation of pseudomembrane. Lichen planus causes erythematous lesions where Wickham striae are present and may in rare cases develop erosions. In most cases of oral lichen planus, these are asymptomatic manifestations with few complications. Even though these diseases show some similarity to PNP, they are less aggressive, lethal, painful, and incapacitating, with less ability to spread to all mucosal and other body sites when compared to PNP [28, 42, 43].

5.2 Secondary mucosal lesions

Lesions can also affect regions such as the oropharynx, esophagus, stomach, duodenum, large intestine, conjunctiva, and anogenital region [2, 3, 7, 39, 41, 44, 45]. The involvement of the oropharynx and esophagus commonly triggers painful sensations and dysphagia [4]. The anogenital lesions demonstrate red-violet erythema in the glans or its surroundings (**Figure 2**). In some cases, lichen planus presents a possible differential diagnosis. However, unlike red-violet lesions, lichen planus forms linear white streaks that may arise in the glans, scrotum, and vulva, in addition to the presence of dyspareunia and pruritus [43]. In these patients, both necrosis and loss of epidermis are absent, unlike patients with PNP who present this clinical [43].

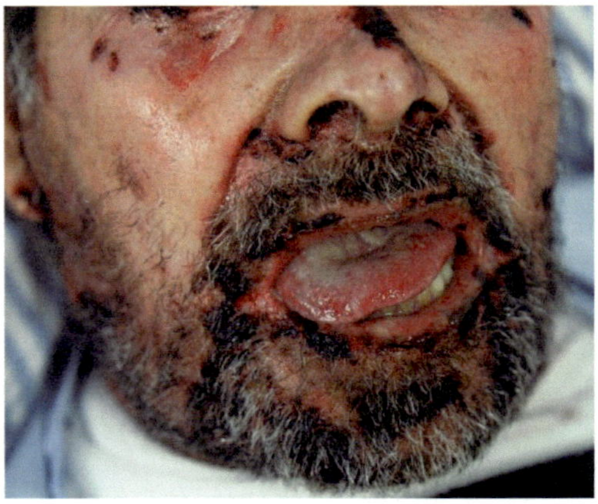

Figure 1.
Severe erosive mucositis with hematic crusting on the lips and oral mucosa.

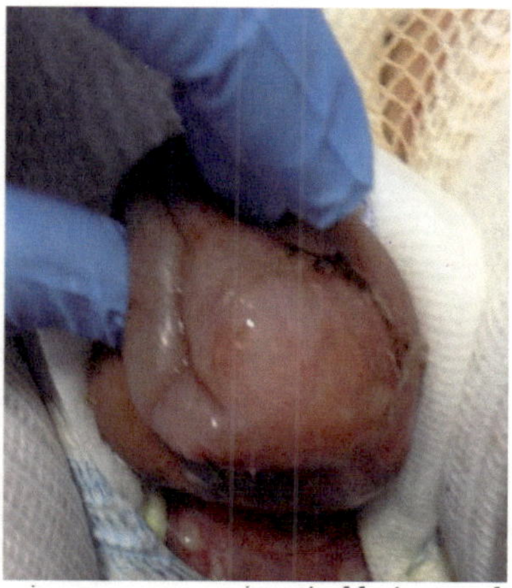

Figure 2.
Red-violet lesion in the genital organ.

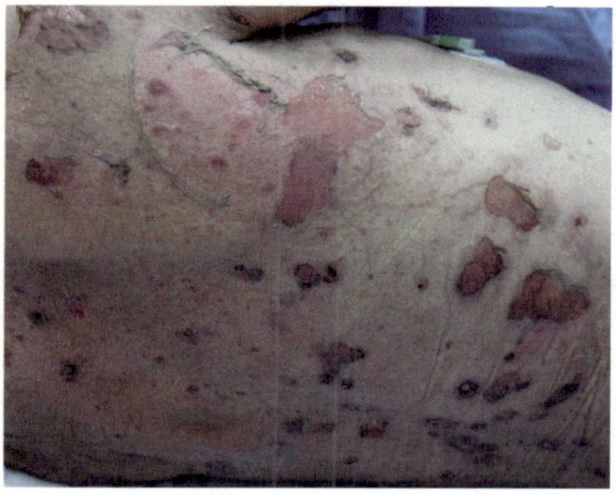

Figure 3.
Extensive erosions and blisters in the dorsal region.

About 70% of the patients present conjunctival lesions such as bilateral bulbar conjunctival hyperemia, diffuse papillary tarsal conjunctival reactions, conjunctival epithelium desquamation, forniceal shortening, painful ocular irritation, poor vision, conjunctival and corneal erosions, and pseudomembranous conjunctivitis [2, 46, 47].

5.3 Skin lesions

Skin lesions usually appear soon after the onset of mucosal involvement [48]. The most affected sites are the dorsal region (**Figure 3**), head, and neck (**Figure 4**), in addition to the nearby extremities [4, 39, 49]. Patients with PNP started the study in very different ways, with the first signs being erythema, bullous and vesicular lesions, papules, skin scaling with Nikolsky sign, exfoliative erythema, and ulcers with hematic crust. Often, the first clinical sign on the skin is erythema that may progress with bullous and ulcerated lesions [24, 50]. Unlike adults, PNP in the skin of children appears in the form of lichenoid lesions, rather than bullous lesions.

Similar to PNP, bullous pemphigoid (BP) provides blistering with erythematous base or normal skin. However, BP lesions occur more frequently in the lower abdomen and lower limbs, and in most individuals, mucosal lesions are not affected [51]. In addition, pruritus is present in the vast majority of these patients, unlike PNP, which show painful and disseminated lesions mainly in the upper body and mucosal regions [28, 51].

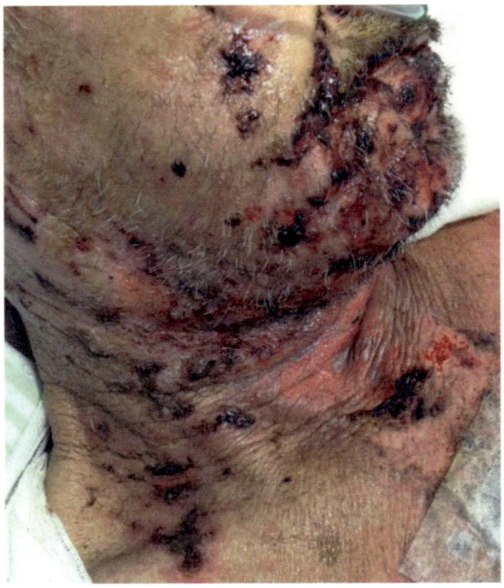

Figure 4.
Confluent erosions with hematic crusts in the head and neck region.

Already erythema multiforme shows prodromal symptoms such as fever and myalgia before the appearance of lesions on the mucosal and skin. Their skin lesions change in feature according to the course of the disease and resemble insect bites or hives that result in the well-known targetoid lesions that are common in this disease. Although cases of necrosis and blisters occur in the center of the lesions, this disease shows less aggression and fewer blisters and ulcers with hematic crusts than the patients affected by PNP [42].

Lichen planus affects flexor surfaces of the wrists, forearm, and legs. These lesions have round reticular white lines such as Wickham striae. They may arise in places that suffer trauma (Koebner's phenomenon), in addition to making the site pigmented after inflation, thus demonstrating clinical differences in cutaneous erosions seen in the course of PNP progression [43].

The graft versus host disease causes rash and maculopapular rash that present itching and can spread to the entire body, less in the scalp. In very severe cases, there may be some sites with necrosis at the base of epidermal rete pegs [52]. Generally, these severe cases are differentiated from the PNP both by the patient's clinical history and by skin biopsy that demonstrate distinct histopathological characteristics.

5.4 Pulmonary manifestations

Approximately 92.8% of the cases described in the literature show pulmonary involvement [3]. The pulmonary clinical signs of PNP are dyspnea, obstructive pulmonary disease, and bronchiolitis obliterans. The resolution of pulmonary problems is of extreme importance, since it is the main cause of death in individuals with PNP [53]. The patients with the greatest pulmonary involvement are Chinese children and patients with Castleman disease [53]. Studies show that 71% of the patients had bronchiolitis obliterans organizing pneumonia, and they give worse prognosis even if treatment of the neoplasia occurs [12, 54].

6. Histopathological examination

The pathological analyses demonstrate many varied aspects, since they show them peculiar characteristics according to the evaluated lesions [55]. When

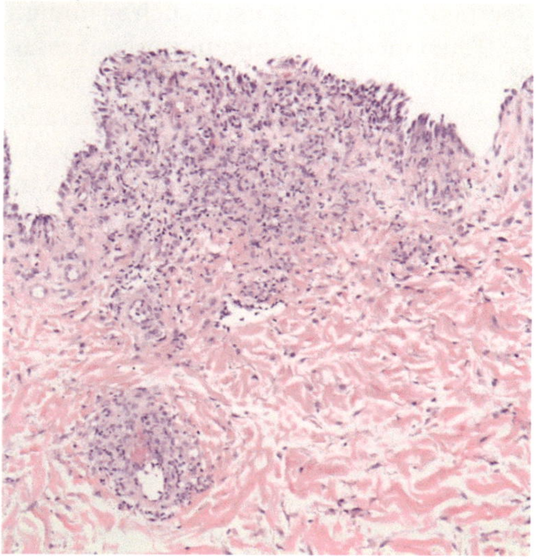

Figure 5.
Histopathological examination of the biopsy specimen showing keratinocyte apoptosis and acantholysis (hematoxylin and eosin, original magnification × 100).

analyzing the biopsy of blisters, we found acantholysis with inflammatory infiltrates (**Figure 5**) [55]. However, when it presents inflammatory maculopapular lesions, the most common findings are lichenoid interface dermatitis [55]. In the presence of lesions with the presence of blisters and maculopapular lesions, mixed characteristics of each type of lesion may occur in the pathology. The findings with dyskeratosis and suprabasal acantholysis are one of the most important characteristics that lead to the definitive diagnosis of PNP [6]. Dyskeratosis is an abnormal formation of epidermal keratinization, whereas acantholysis is the loss of adhesion between skin cells [28]. These findings may help in the diagnosis even when there is no possibility of performing direct immunofluorescence (DIF) or when they are negative [39, 55]. DIF is a laboratory technique capable of detecting the deposition of autoantibodies and immune cells in the sites affected by the disease. The use of DIF demonstrates an extremely important technique for the diagnosis of PNP, since it can analyze both specific autoantibodies and cytotoxic cells of the human immune system, such as CD8+ T cells that act by attacking several layers with keratin and demonstrating intracellular staining of cementum and/or marking of epidermal dermal junctions in band [28, 55].

7. Immunological studies

The use of DIF demonstrates great importance in the diagnosis of PNP even though approximately 50% of the cases show negative [3]. This technique shows a staining in IgG deposition intracellular chicken wire pattern (linear formation of autoantibodies deposition) along the dermoepidermal junction in both the linear form, as granulate [15]. The presence of IgG deposition in the dermoepidermal region is very characteristic of the PNP; however, only 25% presents this pattern [56].

The use of indirect immunofluorescence (IIF) shows involvement of the epidermis by the deposition of IgG in the intercellular regions. Other techniques used as cytoplasmic fluorescence (intracellular staining) demonstrate a prominent basal staining. IIF marking is extremely strong in the layers of the epithelium, and this, alerting to PNP investigation, since it shows high specificity [56].

Other serological methods may also be used, such as immunoprecipitation, immunoblot and anti-EP enzyme-linked immunosorbent assay (ELISA) [57–59]. Studies evidenced 95 and 100% sensitivity in radioactive and nonradioactive immunoprecipitation techniques, respectively, and this demonstrates that immunoprecipitation is the most serologically sensitive test for PNP diagnosis [57, 60, 61]. Currently the immunoprecipitation is considered gold standard in the diagnosis of PNP, that is, the main criterion to diagnose [62, 63].

8. Diagnosis

The criteria for diagnosis according to Anhalt et al. in 1990 are based on five criteria, such as clinical characteristics, histopathological analysis, direct and indirect immunofluorescence, and immunoprecipitation [1]. These criteria have been modified and adapted. In 1993, researchers included to perform the diagnosis the presence of three main criteria or two major and two minor [63]. Already in 2002, Mimouni et al. reviewed the Anhalt criteria and considered four minimum criteria of high confidence in diagnosis (**Table 2**) [12]. DIF is a nonessential criterion because of its low sensitivity. As for IIF on rat bladder epithelia and monkey esophagus, they were considered useful for tracking and detecting PNP [57, 64]. Negative IIF cannot exclude PNP, and other techniques such as immunoblotting and immunoprecipitation should be used to confirm or rule out a diagnosis.

1. Clinical features of severe and protracted mucosal involvement and polymorphic cutaneous eruptions
2. Histologic features of acantholysis or lichenoid or interface dermatitis
3. Demonstration of antiplakin autoantibodies
4. The presence of an underlying neoplasm, especially lymphoproliferative tumors

Table 2.
Minimum criteria for diagnosis.

9. Differential diagnosis

The diagnosis of PNP can be complex and difficult to perform because there are several similar diseases (**Table 3**). PNP and pemphigus vulgaris (PV) are very similar clinically, but some details differentiate them. PNP develops with inflammatory papules or macules that progress to blisters, while PV presents bullous lesions with a reddish background. Molecularly, the PNP presents some antibodies specific for this disease, such as the presence of anti-A2ML1, anti-envoplakin, and anti-periplakin, and demonstrates patterns of IgG deposition on cell surfaces with accumulation in the basement membrane zone [57, 64–66]. Even though bullous autoimmune diseases resemble each other, PNP differentiates it by the presence of antibody that stains the mouse bladder. In bullous pemphigoid (PB), BP230 and BP180 can be found, as well as in PNP. However, the use of DIF differentiates them by the IgG deposition patterns found in the PNP. The involvement by morbilliform-like erythema, toxic epidermal necrolysis, and Stevens-Johnson syndrome can also be confused with PNP. However, the detection of antibodies, pathological analysis of the lesions, and the patient's clinic can differentiate these diseases [1, 10, 39, 57, 64–66].

Despite some cases that both clinically and histologically resemble each other, it is important to perform other techniques to rule out differential diagnoses. The use of otorhinolaryngological examination is very important to differentiate the diseases

Disease	Causers	Pathophysiology
Pemphigus vulgaris	Autoimmune reaction	Autoantigens anti-desmoglein 1,3
Bullous pemphigoid	Autoimmune reaction	Autoantigens anti-BP180 and anti-BP230
Lichen planus	Autoimmune reaction	Autoantigens anti-keratinocyte and antinuclear
Erythema multiforme	hypersensitivity by infection, viruses and drugs	Infiltration of cytotoxic T cell and increased tumor necrosis factor-α
Toxic epidermal necrolysis	Drug reaction that affects more than 30% of the body	Infiltration of cytotoxic T cell, natural killer, and increased granulysin
Stevens-Johnson syndrome	Drug reaction that affects less than 10% of the body	Infiltration of cytotoxic T cell, natural killer, and increased granulysin
Drug eruption	Drug reaction	Perivascular infiltration by lymphocytes, eosinophils, and increased histamine and leukotrienes

Table 3.
Differential diagnosis.

that affect the mucous membranes. Well-done physical examination of the oral cavity, histopathological analysis characteristics, cutaneous involvement, and the presence of IIF strongly suggest for the diagnosis of PNP [40, 44, 67].

10. Treatment

Effective treatment for PNP is still a major puzzle because of its rarity. Although several drugs are used in the literature, PNP has shown great resistance when compared to other forms of pemphigus [50, 68]. When there is suspicion or evidence of PNP, the performance of the six steps described on 2011 by Frew et al. may provide better management of individuals (**Table 4**) [69]. Stabilization of patients, according to the first step, is the most important step, since it is the major cause of death in patients [69].

Currently, the first-line treatment for PNP is still high doses of corticosteroids [70]. This treatment improves the cutaneous lesions, but the mucosal involvement is little altered. The use of other drugs also shows little efficacy in the lesions of the mucosa, this resistance being the characteristic of the disease [69, 71].

Several studies have shown that the combination of drugs has been effective and safe. These associations were prednisolone used with other therapies, such as mycophenolate mofetil, cyclosporine A, azathioprine, plasmapheresis, and intravenous immunoglobulin [72–77]. Even though treatment is more effective, mucosal involvement is still resistant to such combined therapies [71].

The use of monoclonal antibody has been effective in the treatment of PNP in some case reports described in the literature. Administration of rituximab, an anti-CD20, has shown good PNP therapy due to B-cell lymphoma [78, 79]. This therapy is based on an infusion of 375 mg/m^2 weekly for 4 weeks followed by eight weekly infusions for 4 weeks of corticosteroid and administration of other immunosuppressive drugs such as cyclosporine A [69].

The use of alemtuzumab, a humanized monoclonal antibody that binds to CD52, has been reported. Reported in the treatment of PNP remission in patients whose presence of chronic lymphoid leukemia [80]. Alemtuzumab has been used in a patient with resistance to other drugs such as corticosteroids, intravenous immunoglobulin,

1. Stabilization of vital parameters
2. Assessment of any underlying malignancy
3. Diagnosis of PNP
4. Removal and therapy for the triggering tumor
5. Treatment of PNP

Table 4.
Management of the patient with suspected PNP.

and cyclosporine A. In this patient, intravenous 30 mg was infused three times a week for 3 months. Even though there was improvement in both skin and mucosal lesions, the patient continued maintenance treatment with 500 mg of mycophenolate mofetil and 5 mg of prednisone [80]. Although there are several treatment alternatives, new therapies that reduce the resistance of PNP to drugs are still fundamental. Daclizumab, a monoclonal antibody against T-cell interleukin-2, has been shown to be a promising therapy [81].

It is known that in order to avoid large amounts of autoantibodies released into the bloodstream during tumor excision surgery, it is necessary to block blood flow and prevent compression of neoplastic tissue. In addition, the use of intravenous immunoglobulin before and during operations has demonstrated a significant reduction in mortality caused by bronchiolitis obliterans. Even after complete tumor resolution, immunoglobulin administration is required until 2 years to provide remission of autoimmunity triggered by PNP [82, 83].

In addition to the treatment of neoplasia and PNP, other ducts must be performed. When there is loss of skin integrity or immunosuppression, antimicrobial therapy is recommended early to prevent sepsis. Medications for pain control are also useful, since patients have pain in regions with ulceration and erosions [50].

Although there are several treatments stipulated in the literature, there are still no known drugs that reduce the mortality of patients, since the PNP proves highly resistant to more aggressive therapies. However, it is known that management, diagnosis, and early treatment are indispensable methods for a better response of the patients in the prescribed procedures.

11. Prognosis

The prognosis of PNP is extremely poor. Mortality can reach 90% of the cases in the first year, 41% of mortality in the second year, and 38% of death in the third year with the disease [84]. Commonly, death is triggered by systemic complications such as bronchiolitis obliterans, sepsis, and bleeding in the gastrointestinal tract [6, 50]. It is known that regardless of the cure or control of the neoplasia, the PNP progresses, demonstrating itself autonomous to the triggering factor [6, 10, 11, 13, 50]. Patients who exhibit morbilliform erythema and necrosis of skin biopsy keratinocytes demonstrate a worse overall survival [84]. In some cases, the removal of Castleman disease and benign thymoma has shown better results than other underlying diseases [84, 85].

Even with a high mortality rate, the prognosis depends very much on the proper management of the patient, such as monitoring of vital signs, control of oral and skin lesions, treatment of the triggering disease, and prevention of sepsis and bronchitis obliterans. For this, it is essential to follow the patient closely and treat the disease aggressively [50].

12. Quality of life

Studies have mentioned severe losses in the quality of life of patients with pemphigus. The main criteria that impair the quality of life were the greater severity of the disease, anxiety, and depression. However, there was no clear measurement of gender, age, type of pemphigus, duration of disease, skin involvement, disease activity, itching, burning sensation in the skin, or treatment in use [86]. There is still a great need in the standardization and validation of PNP-specific questionnaires, as this proves to be extremely important in order to know and enable actions at key points by multidisciplinary teams.

13. Conclusions

PNP demonstrates a great challenge for physicians, since it presents several clinical aspects and varied degrees of bodily involvement. Early diagnosis, management of the patient, treatment of the underlying neoplasia, and aggressive treatment for PNP are of paramount importance for the best prognosis of the patient, since it is an extremely lethal disease. For this, more studies are needed to better understand the disease and cooperation between multidisciplinary teams involving dermatologists, oncologists, hematologists, otorhinolaryngologists, surgeons, ophthalmologists, immunologists, psychologists, nurses, and social workers.

Acknowledgements

The author would like to acknowledge the help of Dr. Paulo Prata and the School of Health Sciences Barretos, São Paulo, Brazil.

Conflict of interest

The author has declared no conflicts of interest.

Appendices and nomenclature

A2ML1	alpha-2 macroglobulin-like 1
BP	bullous pemphigoid
DIF	direct immunofluorescence
DSG	desmoglein
IIF	indirect immunofluorescence
LPD	lymphoproliferative disorders
PNP	paraneoplastic pemphigus

Author details

Richard Lucas Konichi-Dias
School of Health Sciences, Dr. Paulo Prata-FACISB, Barretos, Sao Paulo, Brazil

*Address all correspondence to: richardkonichi95@gmail.com

References

[1] Anhalt GJ, Kim SC, Stanley JR, et al. Paraneoplastic pemphigus. An autoimmune mucocutaneous disease associated with neoplasia. The New England Journal of Medicine. 1990;**323**:1729-1735

[2] Nguyen VT, Ndoye A, Bassler KD, et al. Classification, clinical manifestations, and immunopathological mechanisms of the epithelial variant of paraneoplastic autoimmune multiorgan syndrome: A reappraisal of paraneoplastic pemphigus. Archives of Dermatology. 2001;**137**:193-206

[3] Paolino G, Didona D, Magliulo G, et al. Paraneoplastic pemphigus: Insight into the autoimmune pathogenesis, clinical features and therapy. International Journal of Molecular Sciences. 2017;**18**:2532. DOI: 10.3390/ijms18122532

[4] Anhalt GJ. Paraneoplastic pemphigus. The Journal of Investigative Dermatology. Symposium Proceedings. 2004;**9**:29-33

[5] Sinha AA. Paraneoplastic pemphigus: Autoimmune-cancer nexus in the skin. Anti-Cancer Agents in Medicinal Chemistry. 2015;**15**:1215-1223

[6] Vassileva S, Drenovska K, Manuelyan K. Autoimmune blistering dermatoses as systemic diseases. Clinics in Dermatology. 2014;**32**:364-375

[7] Czernik A, Camilleri M, Pittelkow MR, et al. Paraneoplastic autoimmune multiorgan syndrome: 20 years after. International Journal of Dermatology. 2011;**50**:905-914

[8] Sticherling M, Erfurt-Berge C. Autoimmune blistering diseases of the skin. Autoimmunity Reviews. 2012;**11**:226-230

[9] Pollmann R, Schmidt T, Eming R, et al. Pemphigus: A comprehensive review on pathogenesis, clinical presentation and novel therapeutic approaches. Clinical Reviews in Allergy and Immunology. 2018;**54**:1-25

[10] Sehgal VN, Srivastava G. Paraneoplastic pemphigus/paraneoplastic autoimmune multiorgan syndrome. International Journal of Dermatology. 2009;**48**:162-169

[11] Cervini AB, Tosi V, Kim SH, et al. Paraneoplastic pemphigus or paraneoplastic autoimmune multiorgan syndrome. Report of 2 cases in children and a review of the literature. Actas Dermo-Sifiliográficas. 2010;**101**:879-886

[12] Mimouni D, Anhalt GJ, Lazarova Z, et al. Paraneoplastic pemphigus in children and adolescents. British Journal of Dermatology. 2002;**147**:725-732

[13] Lane JE, Woody C, Davis LS, et al. Paraneoplastic autoimmune multiorgan syndrome (paraneoplastic pemphigus) in a child: Case report and review of the literature. Pediatrics. 2004;**114**:e513-e516

[14] Geller S, Gat A, Harel A, et al. Childhood pemphigus foliaceus with exclusive immunoglobulin G autoantibodies to desmocollins. Pediatric Dermatology. 2016;**33**:e10-e13

[15] Amber KT, Valdebran M, Grando SA. Paraneoplastic autoimmune multiorgan syndrome (PAMS): Beyond the single phenotype of paraneoplastic pemphigus. Autoimmunity Reviews. 2018;**17**:1002-1010

[16] Kaplan I, Hodak E, Ackerman L, et al. Neoplasms associated with paraneoplastic pemphigus: A review with emphasis on non-hematologic malignancy and oral mucosal manifestations. Oral Oncology. 2004;**40**:553-562

[17] Shahidi-Dadras M, Abdollahimajd F, Barzkar N, et al. Paraneoplastic pemphigus with underlying retroperitoneal inflammatory myofibroblastic tumor: A case report and review of the literature. Indian Dermatology Online Journal. 2017;**8**:478-481

[18] Lim JM, Lee SE, Seo J, et al. Paraneoplastic pemphigus associated with a malignant thymoma: A case of persistent and refractory oral ulcerations following thymectomy. Annals of Dermatology. 2017;**29**:219-222

[19] Cho JH, Kim NJ, Ko SM, et al. A case report of paraneoplastic pemphigus associated with esophageal squamous cell carcinoma. Cancer Research and Treatment. 2013;**45**:70-73

[20] Wang Y-Z, Gao Z-Y, Lei F-M, et al. A case report on paraneoplastic pemphigus associated colonic carcinoma. Chinese Medical Journal. 2016;**129**:1501-1502

[21] Gill H, Trendell-Smith NJ, Loong F, et al. Paraneoplastic pemphigus due to CD8-positive cytotoxic T-cell lymphoma. British Journal of Haematology. 2010;**149**:464

[22] Ghigliotti G, Di Zenzo G, Cozzani E, et al. Paraneoplastic autoimmune multi-organ syndrome: Association with retroperitoneal Kaposi's sarcoma. Acta Dermato-Venereologica. 2016;**96**:261-262

[23] Hong WJ, Lee SE, Chang S-E, et al. Paraneoplastic pemphigus associated with metastatic lymphoepithelioma-like carcinoma originating from the thyroid gland. The British Journal of Dermatology. 2015;**172**:831-834

[24] Ohzono A, Sogame R, Li X, et al. Clinical and immunological findings in 104 cases of paraneoplastic pemphigus. The British Journal of Dermatology. 2015;**173**:1447-1452

[25] Verrini A, Cannata G, Cozzani E, et al. A patient with immunological features of paraneoplastic pemphigus in the absence of a detectable malignancy. Acta Dermato-Venereologica. 2002;**82**:382-384

[26] Liu Q, Bu D-F, Li D, et al. Genotyping of HLA-I and HLA-II alleles in Chinese patients with paraneoplastic pemphigus. The British Journal of Dermatology. 2008;**158**:587-591

[27] Martel P, Loiseau P, Joly P, et al. Paraneoplastic pemphigus is associated with the DRB1*03 allele. Journal of Autoimmunity. 2003;**20**:91-95

[28] Kasperkiewicz M, Ellebrecht CT, Takahashi H, et al. Pemphigus. Nature Reviews Disease Primers. 2017;**3**:17026

[29] Okahashi K, Oiso N, Ishii N, et al. Paraneoplastic pemphigus associated with Castleman disease: Progression from mucous to mucocutaneous lesions with epitope-spreading phenomena. The British Journal of Dermatology. 2017;**176**:1406-1409

[30] Gloghini A, Colombatti A, Bressan G, et al. Basement membrane components in lymphoid follicles: Immunohistochemical demonstration and relationship to the follicular dendritic cell network. Human Pathology. 1989;**20**:1001-1007

[31] Futei Y, Amagai M, Hashimoto T, et al. Conformational epitope mapping and IgG subclass distribution of desmoglein 3 in paraneoplastic pemphigus. Journal of the American Academy of Dermatology. 2003;**49**:1023-1028

[32] Ohyama M, Amagai M, Hashimoto T, et al. Clinical phenotype and anti-desmoglein autoantibody profile in paraneoplastic pemphigus. Journal of the American Academy of Dermatology. 2001;**44**:593-598

[33] Schepens I, Jaunin F, Begre N, et al. The protease inhibitor alpha-2-macroglobulin-like-1 is the p170 antigen recognized by paraneoplastic pemphigus autoantibodies in human. PLoS One. 2010;**5**:e12250

[34] Galliano M-F, Toulza E, Gallinaro H, et al. A novel protease inhibitor of the alpha2-macroglobulin family expressed in the human epidermis. The Journal of Biological Chemistry. 2006;**281**:5780-5789

[35] Wang L, Bu D, Yang Y, et al. Castleman's tumours and production of autoantibody in paraneoplastic pemphigus. Lancet. 2004;**363**:525-531

[36] Wang R, Li J, Wang M, et al. Prevalence of myasthenia gravis and associated autoantibodies in paraneoplastic pemphigus and their correlations with symptoms and prognosis. The British Journal of Dermatology. 2015;**172**:968-975

[37] Wade MS, Black MM. Paraneoplastic pemphigus: A brief update. The Australasian Journal of Dermatology. 2005;**46**:1-8. Quiz 9-10

[38] Reich K, Brinck U, Letschert M, et al. Graft-versus-host disease-like immunophenotype and apoptotic keratinocyte death in paraneoplastic pemphigus. The British Journal of Dermatology. 1999;**141**:739-746

[39] Konichi-Dias RL, Ramos AF, de Almeida Santos Yamashita ME, et al. Paraneoplastic pemphigus associated with chronic lymphocytic leukemia: A case report. Journal of Medical Case Reports. 2018;**12**:252

[40] Kelly S, Schifter M, Fulcher DA, et al. Paraneoplastic pemphigus: Two cases of intra-abdominal malignancy presenting solely as treatment refractory oral ulceration. The Journal of Dermatology. 2015;**42**:300-304

[41] Wieczorek M, Czernik A. Paraneoplastic pemphigus: A short review. Clinical, Cosmetic and Investigational Dermatology. 2016;**9**:291-295

[42] Sokumbi O, Wetter DA. Clinical features, diagnosis, and treatment of erythema multiforme: A review for the practicing dermatologist. International Journal of Dermatology. 2012;**51**:889-902

[43] Usatine RP, Tinitigan M. Diagnosis and treatment of lichen planus. American Family Physician. 2011;**84**:53-60

[44] Healy WJ, Peters S, Nana-Sinkam SP. A middle-aged man presenting with unexplained mucosal erosions and progressive dyspnoea. Case Reports. 2015;**2015**:bcr2014208677

[45] Yokokura H, Demitsu T, Kakurai M, et al. Paraneoplastic pemphigus mimicking erosive mucosal lichen planus associated with primary hepatocellular carcinoma. The Journal of Dermatology. 2006;**33**:842-845

[46] Meyers SJ, Varley GA, Meisler DM, et al. Conjunctival involvement in paraneoplastic pemphigus. American Journal of Ophthalmology. 1992;**114**:621-624

[47] Broussard KC, Leung TG, Moradi A, et al. Autoimmune bullous diseases with skin and eye involvement: Cicatricial pemphigoid, pemphigus vulgaris, and pemphigus paraneoplastica. Clinics in Dermatology. 2016;**34**:205-213

[48] Bialy-Golan A, Brenner S, Anhalt GJ. Paraneoplastic pemphigus: Oral involvement as the sole manifestation. Acta Dermato-Venereologica. 1996;**76**:253-254

[49] Mutasim DF, Pelc NJ, Anhalt GJ. Paraneoplastic pemphigus. Dermatologic Clinics. 1993;**11**:473-481

[50] Yong AA, Tey HL. Paraneoplastic pemphigus. The Australasian Journal of Dermatology. 2013;**54**:241-250

[51] Khandpur S, Verma P. Bullous pemphigoid. Indian Journal of Dermatology, Venereology and Leprology. 2011;**77**:450

[52] Ferrara JLM, Levine JE, Reddy P, et al. Graft-versus-host disease. Lancet. 2009;**373**:1550-1561

[53] Maldonado F, Pittelkow MR, Ryu JH. Constrictive bronchiolitis associated with paraneoplastic autoimmune multi-organ syndrome. Respirology. 2009;**14**:129-133

[54] Mar WA, Glaesser R, Struble K, et al. Paraneoplastic pemphigus with bronchiolitis obliterans in a child. Pediatric Dermatology. 2003;**20**:238-242

[55] Zimmermann J, Bahmer F, Rose C, et al. Clinical and immunopathological spectrum of paraneoplastic pemphigus. Journal der Deutschen Dermatologischen Gesellschaft. 2010;**8**:598-606

[56] Poot AM, Siland J, Jonkman MF, et al. Direct and indirect immunofluorescence staining patterns in the diagnosis of paraneoplastic pemphigus. The British Journal of Dermatology. 2016;**174**:912-915

[57] Joly P, Richard C, Gilbert D, et al. Sensitivity and specificity of clinical, histologic, and immunologic features in the diagnosis of paraneoplastic pemphigus. Journal of the American Academy of Dermatology. 2000;**43**:619-626

[58] Hashimoto T, Amagai M, Ning W, et al. Novel non-radioisotope immunoprecipitation studies indicate involvement of pemphigus vulgaris antigen in paraneoplastic pemphigus. Journal of Dermatological Science. 1998;**17**:132-139

[59] Probst C, Schlumberger W, Stöcker W, et al. Development of ELISA for the specific determination of autoantibodies against envoplakin and periplakin in paraneoplastic pemphigus. Clinica Chimica Acta. 2009;**410**:13-18

[60] Poot AM, Diercks GFH, Kramer D, et al. Laboratory diagnosis of paraneoplastic pemphigus. The British Journal of Dermatology. 2013;**169**:1016-1024

[61] Kelly S, Culican S, Silvestrini RA, et al. Comparative study of five serological assays for the diagnosis of paraneoplastic pemphigus. Pathology. 2015;**47**:58-61

[62] Hashimoto T, Amagai M, Watanabe K, et al. Characterization of paraneoplastic pemphigus autoantigens by immunoblot analysis. The Journal of Investigative Dermatology. 1995;**104**:829-834

[63] Camisa C, Helm TN. Paraneoplastic pemphigus is a distinct neoplasia-induced autoimmune disease. Archives of Dermatology. 1993;**129**:883-886

[64] Helou J, Allbritton J, Anhalt GJ. Accuracy of indirect immunofluorescence testing in the diagnosis of paraneoplastic pemphigus. Journal of the American Academy of Dermatology. 1995;**32**:441-447

[65] Cozzani E, Dal Bello MG, Mastrogiacomo A, et al. Antidesmoplakin antibodies in pemphigus vulgaris. The British Journal of Dermatology. 2006;**154**:624-628

[66] Kazerounian S, Mahoney MG, Uitto J, et al. Envoplakin and periplakin, the paraneoplastic pemphigus antigens, are also recognized by pemphigus foliaceus autoantibodies. The Journal of Investigative Dermatology. 2000;**115**:505-507

[67] van der Waal RI, Pas HH, Anhalt GJ, et al. Paraneoplastic pemphigus as the

presenting symptom of a lymphoma of the tongue. Oral Oncology. 1998;**34**:567-570

[68] Lee SE, Hashimoto T, Kim S-C. No mucosal involvement in a patient with paraneoplastic pemphigus associated with thymoma and myasthenia gravis. The British Journal of Dermatology. 2008;**159**:986-988

[69] Frew JW, Murrell DF. Current management strategies in paraneoplastic pemphigus (paraneoplastic autoimmune multiorgan syndrome). Dermatologic Clinics. 2011;**29**:607-612

[70] Martínez De Pablo MI, Iranzo P, Mascaró JM, et al. Paraneoplastic pemphigus associated with non-Hodgkin B-cell lymphoma and good response to prednisone. Acta Dermato Venereologica. 2005;**85**:233-235

[71] Vezzoli P, Berti E, Marzano AV. Rationale and efficacy for the use of rituximab in paraneoplastic pemphigus. Expert Review of Clinical Immunology. 2008;**4**:351-363

[72] Gergely L, Váróczy L, Vadász G, et al. Successful treatment of B cell chronic lymphocytic leukemia-associated severe paraneoplastic pemphigus with cyclosporin A. Acta Haematologica. 2003;**109**:202-205

[73] Williams JV, Marks JG, Billingsley EM. Use of mycophenolate mofetil in the treatment of paraneoplastic pemphigus. The British Journal of Dermatology. 2000;**142**:506-508

[74] Hertzberg MS, Schifter M, Sullivan J, et al. Paraneoplastic pemphigus in two patients with B-cell non-Hodgkin's lymphoma: Significant responses to cyclophosphamide and prednisolone. American Journal of Hematology. 2000;**63**:105-106

[75] Tan-Lim R, Bystryn JC. Effect of plasmapheresis therapy on circulating levels of pemphigus antibodies. Journal of the American Academy of Dermatology. 1990;**22**:35-40

[76] Izaki S, Yoshizawa Y, Kitamura K, et al. Paraneoplastic pemphigus: Potential therapeutic effect of plasmapheresis. The British Journal of Dermatology. 1996;**134**:987-989

[77] Granata G, Greco A, Iannella G, et al. Posterior reversible encephalopathy syndrome—Insight into pathogenesis, clinical variants and treatment approaches. Autoimmunity Reviews. 2015;**14**:830-836

[78] Hertl M, Zillikens D, Borradori L, et al. Recommendations for the use of rituximab (anti-CD20 antibody) in the treatment of autoimmune bullous skin diseases. Journal der Deutschen Dermatologischen Gesellschaft. 2008;**6**:366-373

[79] Hainsworth JD, Burris HA, Morrissey LH, et al. Rituximab monoclonal antibody as initial systemic therapy for patients with low-grade non-Hodgkin lymphoma. Blood. 2000;**95**:3052-3056

[80] Hohwy T, Bang K, Steiniche T, et al. Alemtuzumab-induced remission of both severe paraneoplastic pemphigus and leukaemic bone marrow infiltration in a case of treatment-resistant B-cell chronic lymphocytic leukaemia. European Journal of Haematology. 2004;**73**:206-209

[81] Lee SE, Kim S-C. Paraneoplastic pemphigus. Dermatologica Sinica. 2010;**28**:1-14

[82] Zhu X, Zhang B. Paraneoplastic pemphigus. The Journal of Dermatology. 2007;**34**:503-511

[83] Anhalt GJ. Paraneoplastic pemphigus. Advances in Dermatology. 1997;**12**:77-96. Discussion 97

[84] Leger S, Picard D, Ingen-Housz-Oro S, et al. Prognostic factors of paraneoplastic pemphigus. Archives of Dermatology. 2012;**148**:1165-1172

[85] Wang J, Zhu X, Li R, et al. Paraneoplastic pemphigus associated with castleman tumor: A commonly reported subtype of paraneoplastic pemphigus in China. Archives of Dermatology. 2005;**141**:1285-1293

[86] Rencz F, Gulácsi L, Tamási B, et al. Health-related quality of life and its determinants in pemphigus: A systematic review and meta-analysis. The British Journal of Dermatology. 2015;**173**:1076-1080